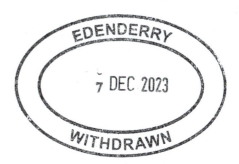

LIFE AT HOME FOR PEOPLE WITH A DEMENTIA

Life at Home for People with a Dementia provides an evidence-based and readable account of improving life at home for people with a dementia and their families. There are estimated to be 47 million people with a dementia worldwide, the majority of whom will live, or want to live, in their own home. Yet there is a major shortcoming in available knowledge on what life is like for people with a dementia living at home. Most research focuses on care in hospitals or care homes, and takes a medical perspective. This book bridges this gap in knowledge by providing a comprehensive and critical overview of the best available evidence on enabling people with a dementia to live well at home from the viewpoint of those living with the condition, and in the context of global policy drivers on ageing and health, as well as technological advances.

The book includes chapters on citizenships – that is, the diversity of people living with a dementia – enabling life at home, rethinking self-management, the ethics and care of people with a dementia at home, technological care and citizenship, and sharing responsibilities. It concludes with a care manifesto in which we set out a vision for improving life at home for people with a dementia that covers the areas of professional practice, education and care research.

By covering a wide range of interrelated topics to advance understanding and practice as to how people with a dementia from diverse backgrounds can be supported to live well at home, this book provides a synthesised, critical and readable understanding of the complexities and risks involved.

Ruth Bartlett is Associate Professor in the School of Health Sciences, University of Southampton, UK, and Director of the University's Dementia Care Doctoral Training Centre. Ruth's research interests are cross-disciplinary and related to people with a dementia, health activism, ageing and participatory research methods, including diary method. Ruth has published academic work and led social research studies in these areas, including most recently a project funded by the Alzheimer's Society on the use of GPS location technologies by people with a dementia and their families.

Tula Brannelly is Lecturer in the School of Health and Social Sciences at Bournemouth University, UK. Tula has a longstanding interest in the experiences of people with a dementia, and has spent many years in research, education and practice. Tula's interest is in the impacts of health and social policy and is informed by an ethics of care. Tula is interested to understand more about how citizenship and care are facilitated with people with a dementia.

LIFE AT HOME FOR PEOPLE WITH A DEMENTIA

Ruth Bartlett and Tula Brannelly

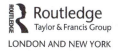
Routledge
Taylor & Francis Group

LONDON AND NEW YORK

First published 2019
by Routledge
2 Park Square, Milton Park, Abingdon, Oxon OX14 4RN

and by Routledge
711 Third Avenue, New York, NY 10017

Routledge is an imprint of the Taylor & Francis Group, an informa business

British Library Cataloguing-in-Publication Data
A catalogue record for this book is available from the British Library

Library of Congress Cataloging-in-Publication Data
Names: Bartlett, Ruth, 1965- author. | Brannelly, Tula, author.
Title: Life at home for people with a dementia / Ruth Bartlett and Tula Brannelly.
Description: Milton Park, Abingdon, Oxon; New York, NY: Routledge, 2018. | Includes bibliographical references and index.
Identifiers: LCCN 2018005054 | ISBN 9781138084742 (hbk) | ISBN 9781138084780 (pbk) | ISBN 9781315111650 (ebk)
Subjects: LCSH: Dementia–Patients–Home care. | Dementia–Patients–Family relationships. | Caregivers.
Classification: LCC RC521 .B372 2018 | DDC 616.8/31–dc23
LC record available at https://lccn.loc.gov/2018005054

ISBN: 978-1-138-08474-2 (hbk)
ISBN: 978-1-138-08478-0 (pbk)
ISBN: 978-1-315-11165-0 (ebk)

Typeset in Bembo
by Deanta Global Publishing Services, Chennai, India

We would like to dedicate this book to all those we have met living with a dementia who have inspired us to write it. Thank you for your perseverance, insights, citizenship and humour.

CONTENTS

A poem by Atherton Gray   *viii*
Foreword by Jim Mann   *ix*
Acknowledgements   *xii*

1   Introduction   1

PART I
Understanding life at home   **13**

2   Citizenships: The diversity of people living at home   15

3   Enabling life at home   32

4   Rethinking self-management   54

PART II
Towards social justice   **71**

5   Ethics and care for people with a dementia at home   73

6   Technological enhanced care and citizenship   92

7   Sharing responsibilities   112

8   A care manifesto   128

Index   *137*

A POEM

Alzheimer's Eponymous Ghost

At the front door
In the first smile of Spring
You are the first stopped
By a soft draught of wisteria perfume.

It seems also to summons
The subtle sound of wavering music
And with the first step you identify
The harmonious chorus of the bees.

Scent and sound are energies of the air
But after the attrition of consciousness
The sense of historical self dissolves
Into a hopeless diagnosis.

In that terrain you are an outcast guest
Exhausting the last atoms of identity
Enduring the dwindling voltage to the end
Like the famished vision of Alzheimer's
eponymous ghost

Shocking family and friends with nothing
To understand or share
A dear wife, a son, a daughter
This year a Summer's bride ….

A poem by Atherton Gray

FOREWORD

'Home is where the heart is' is a saying we have all heard. But for people with a dementia I suggest it is more than that.

Home also represents stability. Order. Routine. Because without that we're flailing. Disoriented. Lost.

It is easy to say 'I want to live at home', but not always so easy to put in place effectively, efficiently or, really, helpfully. Why not? Why is care at home for a person with a dementia diagnosis so challenging?

Are expectations too high for quality in-home care for our loved ones with a dementia? Is a caregiver's view of dementia so wildly different from the rest of society? Why do we seem to accept the lowering of the bar of expectations for people living a dementia diagnosis?

To set the stage, let me first share a few numbers. For the 2018 Alzheimer's Awareness Month, the Alzheimer Society of Canada commissioned a survey that found that 46% of Canadians 'would feel ashamed or embarrassed if they had dementia'. And 27% thought their 'life would be over' if they had a dementia.

Thinking specifically of home care, I was surprised and disappointed to read that only 39% would 'offer support for family or friends' who felt able to be open about their dementia diagnosis.

Put together, I wonder if our reluctance to face dementia, understand it better and freely admit our concerns about it cloud our judgement and opinions. Do we too easily dismiss the individual as being old and maybe hard to take care of, leading some to ask, 'Why take the time and effort to make home safe and secure?'

But I'd like to know why not. People with a dementia diagnosis have a right to life. To live life as they did before their diagnosis. And that means to live in their home, in the neighbourhood they know and perhaps surrounded by friends and caring neighbours.

For sure, there may be services needed to be delivered at home, like medical assistance, but should needing assistance disqualify an individual from living the best they can, in the place where they feel the most productive and able?

On the Alzheimer's Society (UK) site I read about their research that shows that '62% of people with dementia who live alone feel lonely compared to 38% of all people with dementia'. While we know that people who have a dementia diagnosis and live alone are at greater risk of social isolation and loneliness, we also recognise that dementia on its own can cause apathy and a withdrawal from socialising.

This recognition has even extended, at the time I wrote this Foreword, to the UK, where a Minister of Loneliness has been appointed. While the Minister's focus is not wholly on people with a dementia, there is recognition that feeling lonely and isolated impacts the health care system, which, I proffer will affect seniors and people living with a diagnosis of a dementia.

And that is what the authors tackle, especially in Chapters one and two.

We like our independence, don't we? We like feeling we're in charge and living at home gives us the sense that we are in control. We can participate as we like, and, above all, it allows us to feel 'normal'.

But, as the authors note, there are limitations.

Home health services are but one ingredient of living at home upon which many will rely. That said, will home care adequately and compassionately serve the person living with a dementia?

Anecdotally, I have heard disturbing reports where home care comes up short. As one person reported after travelling to see her mother,

> I found her sleeping in her own urine, she smelled bad her hair was greasy. She had homecare come into her home twice a day. She was not taking her medication and no one was notified in the family. The evening person came in did the dishes and left with very little interaction with my mother. The morning one cooked her breakfast but I had to run across the street to buy eggs so there was something to make. No mention that my mother did not have breakfast food in house. She had dinners and leftovers as meals on wheels came in every other day.

Is this an extreme case? I'm not certain, but it was a real and devastating situation to the daughter.

Without the proper supports, staying at home and living well with a dementia may be the biggest challenge we will all face. This is discussed in Chapter three.

Is this where the stride in technology is acknowledged and installed? Is it that easy?

Many of us didn't grow up with technology and now look suspiciously at any technological item, especially one that someone wants to install at home, like a sensor. Who will get the information from the sensor? Will that individual – family member, friend or medical professional – have my best interest at heart or at the first sign of a perceived problem will I be removed from my home and enter a long-term care home? Will the smart furniture or the bathroom or kitchen movement sensor rat me out? Will I be reported if I leave the refrigerator door open too long? What if I sleep in, will the sensor tell on me?

As with everything, technology will not work for everyone in every situation as is discussed in Chapter six.

To be fair, technology has its place and can be unobtrusive, such as one system I saw demonstrated called the Wandering Redirect System (http://www.canassist.ca/EN/main/programs/technologies-and-devices/at-home/wandering-redirect-system.html). With a motion-detected computer tablet on a door, should the resident with a dementia consider leaving the home at an inappropriate time, a video or text message will appear and encourage the individual to, for example, return to bed.

This entire discussion brings to mind two words: risk averse. For all of us living at home there is a certain amount of accepted risk. But is that ready acceptance denied when we reach a certain age or when we live with a diagnosis of a dementia? Is that risk talked about with that individual by family or the doctor beforehand or are assumptions, often ill-conceived, automatically made? Because the individual has a dementia, no matter how far along the journey he or she is, it will be determined, possibly without evidence, that they are incapable of living on their own?

The stigma of dementia is a hard intangible to beat and due to this, decisions can be made unilaterally because, the thinking goes, the person is incapable and incompetent. I have read about The Pygmalion Effect and see its application here. It suggests that when a person is diagnosed with a dementia, the bar – the expectations of that individual – is lowered. Automatically. Rather than 'we're in this together' – whether with family or doctor – it often comes down to 'we know better'. We will therefore tell, not ask, you. There will be no thought given to a shared responsibility as discussed in Chapter seven.

Am I completely sold on the idea of staying at home as long as possible? The jury is still out.

I see and acknowledge the very real benefits. But I also first see the need for better education around dementia – living with dementia and delivering care to people living with a dementia – for families and home care workers. Assumptions and biases around dementia need to be parked at the door and not allowed to influence attitudes in the home.

Living at home longer isn't a new concept but it is one that needs to be improved upon and in this day and age, I am confident can be done effectively, efficiently and with heart. Thank you to the authors for encouraging a conversation about this important piece of living well at home with a dementia diagnosis.

Jim Mann
Vancouver, Canada

ACKNOWLEDGEMENTS

We acknowledge the services of Mrs Vicki Fenerty, subject librarian at the University of Southampton, UK, who located and retrieved many of the research papers we have cited and used in this book. We are grateful to the Alzheimer's Society for supporting this work, and in particular, for funding the GPS Safer Walking Study, which has provided so many useful examples. Finally, we wish to thank Dr Elaine Weirsma (Lakehead University, Canada) for providing such helpful comments on draft chapters, often within a short time frame.

1

INTRODUCTION

Life at home for people with a dementia is under the spotlight. More attention is being paid to improving life at home for individuals and families living with a dementia than ever before. One of the main reasons for this is because dementia is having a major impact on households, communities and countries across the world. Dementia, including Alzheimer's disease, is one of the biggest global public health challenges facing our generation. Today, over 35 million people worldwide live with the condition, and this number is expected to double by 2030 and more than triple by 2050 to 115 million (Prince, Prina, & Guerchet, 2013). In this book, we seek to synthesise the research evidence on life at home for people with a dementia, and provide a fresh context for thinking about and researching this important subject.

To begin, we invite you to consider the following questions: what does 'home' mean to you? How much do you know about the day-to-day life at home for people with a dementia? Is it an area of practice and research that you are familiar with, but would like to know more about? Do you wish that more were written about the complexities and challenges of supporting people with a dementia to live at home? Do you think attitudes and expectations about life at home for people with a dementia are changing? Maybe you can imagine a future when care homes become obsolete – or at least, a less standard part of the long-term care system – because services in the community have become so well integrated and established that people with a dementia no longer need to move into a care home. Maybe you cannot understand why care homes are the norm in some countries but not others.

What risks do you to take when it comes to supporting someone with a dementia to live independently at home? Do you wish you could take more risks? What does independence and interdependence at home mean for someone with a dementia? Self-management – that is, taking responsibility for one's own health and well-being – has become a popular principle in care discourse, but is self-management a sustainable and realistic option for a person with a dementia? How can the responsibilities of care and social citizenship be shared? Who should share such responsibilities, and can they ever be completely shared? What are the ethics of sharing responsibilities? What role do technologies have in delivering care and upholding citizenship? Perhaps you envision a world in which the very latest technologies are seamlessly integrated into people's lives? Maybe you have concerns about the ethics and legalities of using certain technologies to support people with a dementia.

How much do you know about the friendships and support networks between people with a dementia and their families? How important do you believe these are for health and well-being and quality of life? Are they essential if a person with a dementia wants to stay at home? What about bodies and the material space people occupy? How much consideration should be given to these matters when decisions are being made about where a person with a dementia lives?

What does it mean to be a 'good citizen' in the 21st century when you have a dementia and are faced with cognitive and sensory challenges? How much say does a person with a dementia have in decisions about their life? How much control does a person have? How much influence and control is it possible to have when you have a dementia? How seriously do you take someone with a dementia? What support do you think people with a dementia need to stay in control? What power do people with a dementia have? How can it be increased? Do you hope for a future when the wishes of people with a dementia are not only listened to but acted upon? Do you wish that people with a dementia had more access to justice?

These are the kind of questions and topics dealt with this in this text. The idea is to start reimagining and reframing life at home for people with a dementia, by reflecting on your responses to these questions. You may have found some questions more challenging than others. Equally some questions may have prompted you to come up with your own. By asking questions it is possible to forge a new meaning about life at home for people with a dementia.

Life at home for people with a dementia

This book is about life at home for people with a dementia and their families in the 21st century. It seeks to provide clarity and a synthesised account of what we know about people with a dementia living in their own homes in the context of discourses of care and citizenship. Discourses of care are essentially about interpersonal relationships while discourses of citizenship are concerned with social justice, which we define as being treated fairly by societal institutions. Drawing simultaneously on these two discourses, we will review and discuss what is known about improving life for men and women with a dementia. The gendered nature of providing and receiving care is a recurring theme. The book is primarily for students, social workers, health care professionals, community workers, researchers, advocates and others interested in enabling people with a dementia to live well at home, including individuals and families living with this condition.

Citizenship is a sensitising concept. It reminds us that people with a dementia are not only 'patients with needs' but persons with a right to experience freedom from discrimination and despair and be regarded as equal members of the socio-political sphere to which they have belonged all their life. Now with the disease, they are still members of and still belong, but in different ways and with different hopes and desires.

The book expands on the understanding people have of life at home for people with a dementia. It prioritises the perspective of people living with a dementia, whilst taking account of the needs and opinions of those around them, including family members and practitioners. Our discussion is based on scholarship from a wide range of disciplines, including citizenship and disability studies, particularly work by feminist scholars, as well as the literature on dementia care, ethics of care, cultural meanings of home, and gerontechnology. Research on the design and use of technologies for independent living and social participation of older people – gerontechnology – is growing and changing the nature of care at home for people with a dementia. Hence, it is timely and important to draw upon this work in this text. The sociological literature on personal lives and family practices is marshalled to provide a normative framework for exploring life at home for people with a dementia. Our intention is to use emancipatory concepts to reframe life at home for people with a dementia.

Our motivation for writing this book is to provide a systematic focus on improving life at home for people living with a dementia. In particular, we want to explore meanings of care and social citizenship to people in this situation. Drawing on the latest research, including our own, we argue that people living with a dementia are *entitled* to live at home – even those individuals with complex care needs who may require round-the-clock support. It is our view that all citizens are entitled to live at home rather than be institutionalised. That is not to say everyone with a dementia *should* live at home, but that people have a right to expect effective measures to be taken to enable them to do so if that is what they wish. We hope this book becomes part of a wider rallying call to move away from the over-development of residential care, towards the deinstitutionalisation of people with a dementia.

In many countries, when life at home becomes too challenging, placement in a nursing home is seen as the answer (Björnsdóttir, Ceci, & Purkis, 2015). The institutionalisation rate of people with a dementia is higher than any other group in society. One systematic review found that it increased from almost 20% in the first year after diagnosis of dementia to around 50% after five years and up to 90% after eight years; in fact, the risk of nursing home placement increased fivefold for people with a dementia compared to people without a dementia (Luppa, Luck, Brähler, König, & Riedel-Heller, 2008). This is neither sustainable nor fair, especially as institutionalisation is associated with increased mortality, restricted quality of life as well as questionable quality of care (Luppa et al., 2009). Nevertheless, institutional care for older people with high care needs remains the cultural norm in most Western societies.

Take, for example, the UK. At the time of writing, a population-based study was reported and the conclusion drawn by the research team is a telling one. The UK-based researchers found that between 1991 and 2011, life expectancy increased in Britain by more than four years for both men and women, to 82.6 and 85.6 respectively. But the number of those years spent with substantial care needs rose much more rapidly, from 1.1 to 2.4 for men and 1.6 to three for women (Kingston et al., 2017). The researchers predicted that by 2025 there will be another 350,000 people in Britain with high care needs. What is striking about this piece is the conclusion drawn at the end, which is that 'further population ageing will require an extra 71215 care home places by 2025' (Kingston et al., 2017). Such forecasting is designed to help with future funding decisions. Nonetheless, it shows how acceptable it is (in the West) to propose more *communal* care for people with 'high care needs', as opposed to improving community-based services. This is in stark contrast to disability studies where deinstitutionalisation messages are ongoing and remain strong (Kelly, 2016).

Another motivation for writing this book, then, is to help reverse the trend towards the over-development of residential care, towards the deinstitutionalisation of people with a dementia. Deinstitutionalisation – that is, the development of community-based services as an alternative for care provided in institutional settings – has become the hallmark strategy of social and care services for individuals with limited autonomy across European countries (Ilinca, Leichsenring, & Rodrigues, 2015). People with a dementia have the right to choose their place of residence and have access to a range of in-home services, including personal assistance necessary to support independent living in the community (Article 19 of the Convention of Rights of Persons with a Disability). Moreover, the care home industry is facing a funding crisis, and so more community-based options need to be available. We hope this book becomes a part of this wider social justice agenda, by providing the language and information that individuals and organisations need to promote care at home.

To compile the book, we spoke directly to various people with experience of life at home with a dementia to bring the work alive. We visited people with a dementia and their family members in their own homes to share and talk about what we were planning to write and to ascertain whether there were any particular topics we should cover. One topic which we had not planned to discuss in this book but have done so because of this process is genetic testing and counselling. We also solicited the views and opinions of family members via email and telephone interviews. Throughout this process, we endeavoured to make it clear to people that we were attempting to assemble relevant information about making life at home liveable for people with a dementia and their family carers. Our mission, therefore, is a pedagogic one, as well as transformative.

We also watched and/or listened to some of the accounts of people living with a dementia, which are publicly available on the internet. An increasing number of men and women with a dementia are using social media platforms to express themselves; many of these individuals (although not all) live at home. Take, for example, Peter Berry who has Alzheimer's disease. Peter began a weekly vlog in June 2017, which at the time of writing this text he was posting on YouTube and tweeting a link to his vlog every Friday from @PeterBe1130. Others are making the most of the new opportunities available designed to 'give voice' to people with a dementia, including, for example, Dementia Diaries (see Box 1.1). These perspectives can help us to understand what life is like for people with a dementia living at home. In particular, they show how new mobile technologies have the potential to improve disability citizenship in the 21st century (Darcy, Maxwell, & Green, 2017).

BOX 1.1 DEMENTIA DIARIES

Dementia Diaries is a UK-wide project that brings together people's diverse experiences of living with a dementia as a series of audio diaries. It serves as a public record and a personal archive that documents the views, reflections and day-to-day lives of people living with a dementia, with the aim of prompting dialogue and changing attitudes. The Dementia Diaries initiative was designed by the non-profit communications agency On Our Radar (www.onourradar.org). It was launched by On Our Radar in January 2015 in partnership with Innovations in Dementia, Ownfone and Comic Relief, and was handed over to Innovations in Dementia in August 2016. Phase two of the project is funded jointly by Comic Relief and BIG Lottery Fund.

As well as gleaning the views of people with experience, we undertook an extensive search of databases and 'sweep' of the internet to locate relevant and up-to-date information about life at home for people with a dementia. A librarian was commissioned to search research databases using search terms derived from the book proposal and chapter outlines, such as 'dementia', 'home', 'home care', 'law', 'ethics', 'technology' and 'citizenship'. The search was conducted in February 2017 and the 120+ journal articles that were found were organised according to chapter headings. Articles included the results of systematic reviews as well as surveys and exploratory qualitative studies. Searching the internet identified a number of highly relevant reports published by charitable organisations (e.g. Alzheimer's Society, Alzheimer's Disease International and Alzheimer's Europe) and research funders (e.g. the National Institute for Health Research and the Economic and Social Research Council). In this book, we draw upon and discuss much of this work to show that there is a wealth of empirical knowledge on improving life at home for people with a dementia.

A particularly rich source of data for this book is a research project we have both been directly involved in – Bartlett as the Principal Investigator and Brannelly as the Project Manager. The aim of the research was to examine the usage and effectiveness of GPS 'location' technologies to promote safer walking from the perspective of people with a dementia, family carers and the police, through a process of participative inquiry – that is, knowledge production based on equitable research relations. The work started in November 2015 and was completed in February 2018; it was funded by the Alzheimer's Society. The project consisted of two sequential phases of data collection, followed by a third co-production phase. Phase one involved focus groups with the police (n=20) and individual interviews with people with a dementia (n=16) and family members (n=16). Phase two employed go-along walking interviews with people with a dementia (n=15) who were using some form of technology, such as a GPS device or phone app, when they went out. The third phase involved an overnight residency with key stakeholders including research participants – the aim of which was to share preliminary findings and co-produce key messages for policymakers. The research was conducted in the south of England and covered urban, semi-urban and rural areas. All the participants with a dementia were living in their own homes. We plan to publish the findings of this research elsewhere; our intention here is to use data from what we will refer to hereon as 'The Safer Walking GPS Project' to illustrate various points about ethics, collaboration and sharing responsibilities. Essentially, it is another way of foregrounding the perspective of people with a dementia.

Finally, as well as drawing on published research studies, we searched the British Library for PhD theses deposited in 2016 and 2017 that related to life at home for people with a dementia. We did this to ensure that our discussion included the thinking of emerging (as well as established) scholars in the field of dementia studies. This body of work is encouraging, as it suggests that the perspective of people with a dementia, particularly younger people with a dementia, is beginning to take centre stage. No doubt other countries have a national repository of PhD theses which we could have searched and perhaps discovered even more work, or a different picture. Nevertheless, the British Library was our initial and only source for this book.

There are three major conceptual threads running through the text. The first is the notion of being 'entitled' to live at home rather than the regulated and communal environment of a care home. Conceptualising life at home for people with a dementia in terms of an entitlement means drawing on ideas from citizenship and disability studies, as well as the human rights and care geography literature, and grasping what all of this means in concrete terms. We know that life at home is not always idyllic; it can be a place of confinement, isolation and even violence. Indeed, many of the examples we give in this book are testimony to that. However, people with a dementia are not hostage to fortune; they can change things to meet their needs, given the right support and attitude from others. Thus, our intention is to use the notion of being 'entitled to live at home' as a way of reframing this topic and promoting the idea of people with a dementia as agentic.

A second major thread running through the book is the notion of 'the materiality of care and social citizenship' – that is, the physical or corporeal aspects of life at home. We are particularly interested in how everyday (digital) technologies and systems, such as ambient assisted living systems, feature in the lives of people with a dementia at home. Hence, Chapter six is devoted to the topic of technological enhanced care and citizenship, and this is where the richest discussions about materiality take place. However, the notion of 'the materiality of care and social citizenship' will permeate the text, so the body and the physical environment in which a person lives, including the objects contained within, are not overlooked.

A third major thread underpinning the text is the 'intersections of care and social citizenship' – that is, recognising the multifaceted nature of peoples' lives, and taking account of the differentiated experiences in a person's life. Multiple identities are the norm in society and yet when a person is diagnosed with a dementia that is the identity that tends to dominate. For example, in studies and reports, the 'dementia' typically frames the analysis and discussion, rather than a person's age, social class, ethnicity or gender. In this text, although our primary focus is people living with a dementia, we recognise that the majority of people with this condition will have other identities and are also likely to have another long-term health condition. We appreciate that gender is beginning to feature in dementia discourse, but what about race and class? In addition, whilst it is encouraging to see so many men and women with a dementia speaking out about their experiences of living with a dementia, questions remain about those who choose not to identify themselves as having a dementia or disability, or who cannot speak due to the severity of their condition. We consider these matters of marginalisation, which we are mindful of as we present the evidence. In sum, three threads underpin this text, namely, entitlement and rights, materiality and marginalisation. Together these threads guide our thinking and serve to knit the chapters together to provide a reframing for life at home for people with a dementia. Central to all of this is the ethics of care.

The ethics of care

The ethics of care developed from the work of Carol Gilligan in the 1980s, who examined different gendered responses to moral problems. She found that women were more focused on consequences, in comparison to Kohlberg's experiment that identified that men were more drawn to implementing rules. Ethics of care has since developed into a political theory, particularly through the work of Joan Tronto (1993; 2013), with an applied focus in health and social care (Barnes, 2012, Sevenhuijsen 1998). Tronto (1993: 103) defined care as follows:

> On the most general level, we suggest that caring be viewed as a species activity that includes everything that we do to maintain, continue and repair our world so that we can live in it as well as possible. That world

includes our bodies, our selves and our environment, all of which we seek to interweave in a complex life sustaining web.

There are several key points to make about ethics of care:

1. Care theorists suggest that humans are fundamentally relational and interdependent. Every person is dependent on care to survive into adulthood, and all people give and receive care. Interdependence is the usual state, rather than dependence and independence. This is important as it challenges the idea that certain groups are burdens on society and that caring is problematic. Rather we think of people as needing each other but being in need at some times more than others and that to care well requires adequate resourcing. So, it is not that care is stressful but that doing it alone can be.
2. Care ethics seeks out marginalisation and looks to promote equality. Recognising who is in need is important and taking responsibility for change is fundamental. Political decisions are made about what care is offered to different groups of people. People who provide care cannot adequately care well as they are often low paid and under-resourced. This is consistent with the feminist origins of care ethics – that recognition is the first step in taking responsibility for making a change that leaves no one in poverty or acute need.
3. Experience is central. Understanding the experiences of people involved in giving and receiving care is key to understanding how to better meet needs and achieve care. Because something provided is called care does not mean that it is care. This particularly challenges the idea that the care receiver is the only one who is able to say that care has been achieved – so responsiveness is key and how people are accommodated to respond is key.
4. Context matters. Care ethics values the messy context of everyday life, and the social interdependencies that sustain it. Tronto (2013) recognises that not having enough time to care in our lives creates tension in fulfilling our caring responsibilities. Knowing how to care is dependent on detailed knowledge of care situations, and this requires care practices to enable that.
5. There is an inverse care ratio. People who need care do not get enough of it, and those who get lots of care are not in need. Consider the 3 x 15-minute calls an older person may get at home in contrast to the executive who has various forms of paid help. So, privilege enables some people to get very high levels of care and leaves others with very little, even though the need is greater.

The ethics of care is referred to throughout the book, and relational care is thought to be essential to providing good care to people with a dementia. In addition to the points above, the *integrity of care* is introduced in Chapter four. The integrity of care can be used to guide and critique practice, to understand whose needs are met (or not) through care processes and to understand whether care has occurred.

Terminology and language use are important. We refer to people with experience of living with dementia throughout the book. People with a diagnosis of dementia are referred to as person/people with a dementia. The 'a' is intentional to create space between the person and the dementia. We recognise that those who have mixed forms of dementia may find this problematic. Elsewhere, people are referred to as people with dementias to highlight that there are many forms of dementia. Alternatively, dementia is referred to as dementia syndrome to clarify the nebulous nature of dementia and its impacts on the individual. We also understand that the word dementia is troublesome for many, who would prefer to directly name the cause of dementia, such as Alzheimer's disease, or to refer to cognitive impairment or memory problems. These preferences and clarification attempts show that there is not one preferred way of describing life with a dementia.

Structure of the book

The book is organised into two parts. The first part provides an understanding of 'Life at home' and includes three chapters. Chapter two is on citizenships, and specifically the diversity of people living at home; the word citizenship is pluralised to empathise the myriad of identities and intersections in a person's life. The heterogeneity of people with a dementia will be explored through real-life stories of people with a dementia. Each story is carefully selected and crafted to illustrate the point about the multiple practices of care and social citizenship, and differential experiences of people with a dementia. Through these personal stories, it is possible to highlight the cultural meanings of home, and how different forms of care can challenge or underpin these. The stories also serve to show the diversity of neighbourhoods that people with a dementia are living in, and the ways in which the social determinants of health affect people with a dementia.

Internationalisation and global citizenship are key drivers in learning. Ideas, expressions and care practices from other cultures will therefore be introduced and used to help rethink life at home for people with a dementia. For example, whānau – a Maori term – refers to the broad circle of friends, neighbours and family that can help people at home. Also, the deployment of migrant care workers and domestic maids across Europe and Southeast Asia to provide 24/7 care in the home will be highlighted and discussed, as will research on life at home for people with a dementia from diverse ethnic backgrounds – all of which will broaden understanding of the notion of citizenships and ways of being cared for, and of caring.

The third chapter is about enabling people with a dementia to live at home. There is a growing body of academic literature, practical knowledge and unpublished reports on the experiences of people with a dementia living at home, much of which includes valuable information about what people need to stay at home. However, this work is often 'tucked away' on databases and not shared with those working in the field in a way that is understandable. One of the main aims of this book, and what we intend to do in this chapter, is to distil and organise this evidence. The chapter is organised around four different forms or levels of enabling care and citizenship. These are relational ('who'), service-led ('what'), environmental/geographical ('where') and structural ('how'). Together these enablers form the infrastructure that is required for someone to live at home. These include, for example, cultural values, public policies, social structures and meta narratives about how families 'should' take care of someone with a dementia; meso-enablers, such as service provision, local infrastructure and community resilience; and micro-enablers, such as interpersonal dynamics, impairment effects and personal resources, including resilience. The extent to which services are integrated and meeting people's needs will form a major part of the discussion, as will the importance of rethinking the nature of service provision. There is also a growing policy emphasis on the need to slow the progression of the disease with the costs of caring for people increasing as the condition becomes more severe (Alzheimer's Research UK, 2014).

Chapter four is about self-management. As already mentioned, self-management involves taking responsibility for one's own health and well-being, and is increasingly seen as a key to helping people stay at home. However, rethinking life at home for people with a dementia requires rethinking our notion of self-management. In this chapter, we discuss the idea of self-management and consider what it means in relation to people with a dementia. The concept of self-management has become popular in the policies and practice of many Western societies, where independence, autonomy and being able to look after yourself are held in high regard. In a sense, self-management has become the panacea for unjust health care.

Self-management is about someone with a health condition maintaining themselves and staying well for as long as they possibly can. It requires a person to understand and manage their own condition and treatment, and to know when and who to ask for help. Conventionally, self-management includes some level of self-monitoring and treatment with medication, as is the case with someone diagnosed with diabetes. However, it is increasingly used to describe a broad spectrum of activities that a person might engage in to stay well, such as taking physical exercise to manage a mental illness.

In this chapter, we aim to apply the idea of self-management to people with a dementia living at home, and suggest that it requires a relational component to be meaningful for this group. This is because, while self-care may be an achievable and desirable aim for some people with a dementia, it will not be possible for everyone, all of the time. As the condition progresses and the effects of dementia become more severe, the ability to self-manage will become more and more precarious and eventually impossible. This chapter deconstructs the concept of self-management in relation to people with a dementia and develops an understanding that is more relational in quality. In developing this new way of thinking about self-management, we examine who needs to be involved, rather than what needs to be done, in order for people with a dementia to live well. Furthermore, we draw on ideas from Eastern cultures, where collectivism and mutualism have more currency than autonomy.

The second part of the book takes the topic of life at home towards a social justice agenda. It includes three chapters, all of which explore how care and social citizenships at home might be realised. Chapter five is about ethical and legal matters. The focus here is on the domestic space – the home – and how it can become politicised, as individuals and families develop ways of dealing with the effects of dementia. Current understandings of cognitive impairment tend to overlook the need for trust as a condition of positive relationships, which has led to interventions or advice for carers that, rather than being based on honesty, is based on what we consider to be a flawed concept of 'therapeutic lying'. We discuss this influence in relation to everyday matters such as confounding locks, deterring people from going out, subterfuge (e.g. hiding medication in food), abuse and neglect (possibly due to poor premorbid relationship), and violence and aggression in the home.

Chapter six focuses on the materiality of home life, in particular the role of modern technologies in peoples' lives and the relationships people have with their physical surroundings. We reflect on how everyday (digital) technologies can enhance care and citizenship, and the right of people with a dementia to expect effective measures to be taken to facilitate their personal mobility and social inclusion. Rethinking life at home for people with a dementia requires a radical rethink about technologies, especially surveillance and artificial intelligence. In this chapter, we consider the role of technologies in enabling people to live a life at home and discuss the ways in which technologies are changing the nature of care and citizenship practices. Our focus will be on how modern technologies and platforms such as Smart Homes and Virtual Reality systems can be used to meet the needs and help enable the social citizenship of people with a dementia. The chapter will introduce the reader to current thinking from the field of gerontechnology and explain how the latest advances have the potential to help people to remain at home.

Chapter seven is about sharing responsibilities. Improving life at home for people with a dementia requires an acceptance that responsibilities of care and social citizenship need to be shared. No one individual or family can do it alone; it requires multiple actors and a societal approach for people with a dementia to live well at home. In this chapter, we explain and expand upon this idea, providing examples from across scholarship of how the responsibility of caring for and about people with a dementia at home can be and is shared. The chapter will begin by suggesting that certain shifts in the global policy landscape of dementia, and ageing more broadly, are making way for the idea of shared responsibility to evolve. Most notably the drive to extend user involvement into dementia, and the whole 'Dementia Friendly Communities' (DFC) movement. In the past two decades, we have witnessed a revolution in the way that people with a dementia can participate in the development of policy, practice and research. In particular, the DFC movement has meant that more and more sectors of society, including banks and shopping malls, are playing a role in supporting people with a dementia to live at home. This is one way of sharing responsibility, but there are other spheres, which we outline.

In the final concluding chapter, we explain and present a care manifesto. The manifesto sets out a vision for improving life at home for people with a dementia that covers the areas of professional practice, education and care research. It involves bringing together all the ideas presented in the book and drawing some conclusions about the importance of rethinking life at home. In particular, we summarise our position on the role of material culture, like technologies, and consider the possibility of people staying well without input from formal care services. Together these chapters show how much is known about day-to-day life for people with a dementia living at home, and the complexities of providing care and realising social citizenship.

References

Björnsdóttir, K., Ceci, C., & Purkis, M. E. (2015). The 'right' place to care for older people: Home or institution? *Nursing Inquiry, 22*(1), 64–73. https://doi.org/10.1111/nin.12041

Darcy, S., Maxwell, H., & Green, J. (2017). Disability citizenship and independence through mobile technology? A study exploring adoption and use of a mobile technology platform. *Disability & Society, 7599*(March), 1–23. https://doi.org/10.1080/09687599.2016.1179172

Ilinca, S., Leichsenring, K., & Rodrigues, R. (2015). From care in homes to care at home: European experiences with (de)institutionalisation in long-term care (December). Vienna: European Centre for Social Welfare Policy and Research.

Kelly, C. (2016). *Disability Politics and Care: The Challenge of Direct Funding.* Vancouver: University of British Columbia.

Kingston, A., Wohland, P., Wittenberg, R., Robinson, L., Brayne, C., Matthews, F. E., & Weller, R. (2017). Is late-life dependency increasing or not? A comparison of the Cognitive Function and Ageing Studies (CFAS). *The Lancet, 390*(10103), 1676–1684. https://doi.org/10.1016/S0140-6736(17)31575-1

Luppa, M., Luck, T., Brähler, E., König, H. H., & Riedel-Heller, S. G. (2008). Prediction of institutionalisation in dementia: A systematic review. *Dementia and Geriatric Cognitive Disorders, 26*(1), 65–78. https://doi.org/10.1159/000144027

Luppa, M., Luck, T., Weyerer, S., König, H. H., Brähler, E., & Riedel-Heller, S. G. (2009). Prediction of institutionalization in the elderly. A systematic review. *Age and Ageing, 39*(1), 31–38. https://doi.org/10.1093/ageing/afp202

Prince, M., Prina, M., & Guerchet, M. (2013). World Alzheimer report 2013 journey of caring: An analysis of long-term care for dementia (September). London: Alzheimer's Disease International.

PART I
Understanding life at home

2

CITIZENSHIPS

The diversity of people living at home

Introduction

Worldwide, approximately 60% of persons with a dementia live at home. In many countries, people with a dementia are encouraged to live at home for as long as possible, as it is assumed that quality of life is better at home than in institutions (Kerpershoek et al., 2016). Advancing care and citizenship for people with a dementia at home begins by understanding the diversity of this situation. In particular, we need to consider the myriad of ways in which individuals and families respond and adjust to life with a dementia and the diversity of communities in which people currently live and have lived. Previous work has shown that the experiences of dementia are varied, ranging from 'not a big deal' to 'a nuisance' to 'hellish', and are related to privilege and disadvantage (Hulko, 2009: 131). Moreover, dominant discourses of loss have led to the 'de-gendering' of people with a dementia (Sandberg, 2018). Thus, we need to understand life at home in the context of social citizenship – a conceptual lens for examining diversity, belongingness and gender.

Citizenship has multiple meanings. It encompasses a wide range of associations and concepts – from citizenship-as-belonging, citizenship-as-practice to recognition and status, as well as ethics and interpersonal relationships. In fact, 'it is rarely clear what full citizenship entails and herein lies the protean force of the idea of citizenship; it is a never fully realised ideal that always has to be invoked, revisited and discursively reconstructed in order to be effective' (Hansen, 2015: 231). Citizenships is therefore used in this text to evoke a sense of the plurality of meanings and ways that people seek to belong and express themselves and take responsibility for their life.

People with a dementia are differentiated in how they respond to the condition, how they negotiate and access services and how they feel about sharing their experiences. Some people may be reluctant to access services due to their cultural background or may experience services in different ways. Take for example, how one younger aboriginal woman with a dementia described 'feeling out of place' in the Alzheimer's support group because others were much older than her and she was the only person with childcare concerns (O'Connor, Phinney, & Hulko, 2010: 36). Similarly, lesbian, gay, bisexual or transgender (LGBT) people with a dementia may feel as though they do not belong in a traditional support group. Situations like these are a reminder of the importance of taking into account not only gender but also other differences, such as age, ethnicity and sexual orientation, when discussing the lived experience of dementia.

Fundamentally, citizenship involves recognition of the person living with a dementia. Historically, the voices and experiences of people with a dementia have been absent or overshadowed by those of carers. This is apparent from the evidence base where most of our knowledge relates to the experience of family caregivers, particularly the 'caregiver burden'. It is further evidenced by the amount of work related to the attitudes of clinicians and therapists. By evoking the notion of citizenships, we aim to foreground the diverse experiences and voices of people with a dementia and recognise individuals with this condition in their own right. In the following sections, we discuss how the situation is beginning to change, as some citizens with a dementia are being recognised and heard but not all; hence, the need to recognise the various meanings and sites of citizenship.

Working hard, in the public sphere

> *To seize the opportunities offered by illness, we must live illness actively: we must think and talk about it.*
>
> *(Frank, 1995: 3)*

In the last two decades, citizens with a dementia have been seizing the opportunities offered by this condition; many are speaking out in public, talking at conferences, educating medical and health care students, publishing books and memoirs, tweeting and blogging and taking part in the development of national and regional dementia plans. In so doing, they are subverting negative stereotypes about dementia and challenging others to rethink the category 'dementia'. Take for example Wendy Mitchell who was diagnosed with Alzheimer's disease and vascular dementia aged 58. Wendy has recently published a book, *Somebody I Used to Know*, in which she describes how the condition has affected her (Mitchell, 2018). Others have done the same, including Kate Swaffer, a former nurse who was diagnosed with younger-onset aged 49 (Swaffer, 2016), and Christine Bryden, who was diagnosed with Alzheimer's disease at the age of 46 (Bryden, 2005). Some individuals in the UK are choosing to record their experiences through the Dementia Diaries. Thousands of citizens with a dementia across the world are sharing their experiences of living with this condition, in print, online and face-to-face. Every single person is doing an important job.

Sharing one's experiences publicly, of living with a dementia, helps to subvert negative stereotypes associated with this condition. The stereotype 'elderly' is especially strong, as dementia has become a 'byword for the frailties and fears of aging' (ERSO, 2014: 1). Therefore, hearing so many younger people's stories of living with a dementia is no doubt helping to combat this idea. Evidence suggests that people with a dementia can feel stigmatised by the label 'dementia' and are aware of negative ideas held about them (e.g. Bartlett, 2007; Hulko, 2009). Any attempt, therefore, to combat or subvert negative stereotypes by thinking and talking about dementia in a different way is welcomed.

Another negative stereotype strongly associated with dementia is withdrawal. Deeply ingrained in the public psyche is the assumption that having dementia automatically leads to a retreat to the 'private' care sphere. For example, when Kate Swaffer was diagnosed with a dementia she was told to give up her job and to find out about aged care services; instead, she went on to campaign and study for a PhD in the experience of living with a dementia (Pitt, 2017). The voices of women are not always heard in public debate and so alternative responses by women are particularly powerful for subverting negative stereotypes. As feminist scholars explain, 'addressing the public and private spheres has been and continues to be relevant in understanding women's inclusion and exclusion in the conceptualisation, theorising and practice of citizenship' (Maratou-Alipranti & Tastsoglou, 2010: 10). Thus, what happens within the home is core to understanding what happens outside for people with a dementia.

So far, the examples we have given of people speaking out in public have been women, purposefully so, as the majority of activists are men. In Bartlett's campaigning for social change study, which involved 15 activists with a dementia (ten men and five women), at least one of the women who took part in the study was aware that she was in the minority: that there were more men campaigning than women (Bartlett, 2014). This participant thought it was because once 'women get a diagnosis (of dementia), if they're in a married state, and they're still with their husband, a lot of men feel that they should protect and take over and cherish and do this and do that and do the next thing, so really disempowering women to maybe become as actively involved' – a viewpoint that is backed up by empirical research on men's and women's responses to the symptoms of a dementia in their spouses. The study was conducted in the United States and based on interviews with 13 male caregivers and 15 female caregivers (Hayes, Zimmerman, & Boylstein, 2010). The researchers found that 'men's involvement in caring for their wives (with a dementia) affirmed their identity as male protector and provider' (p. 1112). Hence, married women with a dementia are less likely to be speaking out because their husbands are 'protecting' them from the perceived risks of being in the public domain.

Gender aside, public discourse about people with a dementia is changing, certainly in the UK. After years of being seen clinically as 'patients with needs', people with a dementia and their family carers have joined forces with state agencies and third sector organisations (notably the Alzheimer's Society) to improve societal attitudes and care practices. The collaboration has culminated in the establishment of the Dementia Action Alliance and the development of a set of 'Dementia Statements', as outlined in Box 2.1

As it states on the Dementia Action Alliance website, 'Grounded in human rights law, the statements are a rallying call to improve the lives of people with

---

BOX 2.1 THE DEMENTIA STATEMENTS

The Dementia Statements

These statements were developed by people with dementia and their carers in April 2017. The person with dementia is at the centre of these statements. They represent everyone living with any type of dementia regardless of age, stage or severity.

The 'we' used in these statements encompasses people with dementia, their carers, their families, and everyone else affected by dementia.

These rights are enshrined in the Equality Act, Mental Capacity legislation, Health and care legislation and International Human Rights law.

1. We have the right to be recognised as who we are, to make choices about our lives including taking risks, and to contribute to society. Our diagnosis should not define us, nor should we be ashamed of it.
2. We have the right to continue with day-to-day and family life, without discrimination or unfair cost, to be accepted and included in our communities and not live in isolation or loneliness.
3. We have the right to an early and accurate diagnosis, and to receive evidence based, appropriate, compassionate and properly funded care and treatment, from trained people who understand us and how dementia affects us. This must meet our needs, wherever we live.
4. We have the right to be respected, and recognised as partners in care, provided with education, support, services, and training which enables us to plan and make decisions about the future.
5. We have the right to know about and decide if we want to be involved in research that looks at cause, cure and care for dementia and be supported to take part.

Taken from the National Dementia Alliance
website (https://www.dementiaaction.org.uk/)

dementia and to recognise that people should not be treated differently because of their diagnosis'. While these are laudable proclamations, there is no explanation as to *how* we might realise them. Nor how everyday life can 'continue' when there are so many changes brought about by the diagnosis of a dementia. Furthermore, questions remain about the experiences of those who choose not (or who are unable) to speak out and who remain unheard, including, for example, those who are housebound or who have lived with other disabilities or discriminations throughout their life (such as people with a learning disability, or those who are Deaf).

From an inclusive citizenship perspective, it is important to recognise the diversity of people's experiences of living with a dementia, not only those who speak out publicly. One might ask, for example, how are 'quieter' people with a dementia affected by this new generation of vocal citizens with a dementia? Bartlett asked this question of herself, following an event she organised as part of her campaigning study in 2012. The event was open to members of the public and involved people with a dementia speaking publicly about their experiences of campaigning. Afterwards, Bartlett received an email from a woman who had attended with her 82-year-old mother who lived at home and had Alzheimer's disease. She said, 'My mother thought she was doing okay until she saw these other people with a dementia; it has set her back.' Cleary, different people have different ideas of what it means to 'live illness actively'. Additionally, one might ask, what happens if a person with a dementia has severe aphasia and word finding difficulties? Might the pressures of public speaking be too much for these individuals? (How) do the charities and public agencies who create many of the opportunities for people with a dementia to speak in public support them?

Working hard, in the private sphere

> Stories are not material to be analysed but relationships to be entered.
>
> *(Frank, 1994: 25)*

The following stories are about ordinary men and women living with a dementia. At the centre of each story, is a relationship involving a person with a dementia in their 80s, who lives at home. Each person with a dementia we meet is working hard due to the 'cumulative complexities' of having to handle multiple health conditions over an extended period of time (Shippee, Shah, May, Mair, & Montori, 2012: 1041). In addition, the site of struggle for their rights is the home. By sharing these stories, we aim to open up a discussion about relationality, disability and sociocultural diversity. In particular, we want to make visible the care and citizenship that happens within the private sphere.

This story-telling approach is inspired by the work of Arthur Frank – a trained medical sociologist and professor emeritus of sociology at the University of Calgary, where he has taught since 1975 (taken from his website http://www.arthurwfrank. org/). Frank has written extensively about illness narratives, much of which draws on his personal experiences of living with cancer. Frank's work does not focus on people with a dementia per se, but it is relevant to people with this condition. Take, for instance, his notion of 'deeply ill'; a person with a dementia might be described as 'deeply ill' in the sense that the condition is 'lasting and affects virtually all life choices and decisions'; it certainly alters identity (Frank, 1994: 21). The idea of illness narratives is therefore used to frame and structure this section.

A diagnosis of a dementia is a 'biographical disruption' in that the process and experience fundamentally disrupts a person's plans and relationships in the world (Bury, 1982). Arguably more so for people in their 60s, 50s, 40s or younger, as the condition is strongly associated with old age. Take, for example, Katherine's father, who was diagnosed with early-onset Alzheimer at the age of 64, having recently retired from a busy professional job which involved giving talks and dealing with people. As she told us, it has taken him a long time to find his confidence and voice again. See Box 2.2.

BOX 2.2 KATHERINE TELLS US ABOUT HER FATHER'S RESPONSE TO HIS DEMENTIA DIAGNOSIS

My dad would fit into the category of 'working hard in the private sphere'. He was diagnosed with early-onset Alzheimer's at the age of 64, having recently retired from his busy job as a consultant at the local hospital. He struggled to see himself in the diagnosis and seemed quite unaware of the impact the disease had already had on his life. I think he battled with this diagnosis for a while and by the time he accepted it, his condition had progressed quite significantly, affecting his confidence and limiting how much he wanted to put himself forward and to raise his voice. He has always written poetry and he has been working on one poem since his diagnosis about the impact of the diagnosis. He has been editing it over the last 18 months and still some of the words are being tweaked, perhaps as his feelings about the diagnosis change. This is his way of processing his feelings and for him to quietly push his voice out there. He has now asked for us to get this published for him. I've asked him about whether he'd want to share more of his experiences with others perhaps by giving talks – which he used to do a lot of in a professional capacity – but he seems shy about it and not very confident, questioning whether he had anything to say that others would want to hear. He can find it difficult to find the words he's looking for now and to read out loud, and he seems embarrassed by this and avoids drawing attention to himself. I think a local advocacy group at an early stage would have helped him find his voice but sadly, there was nothing available and his digital literacy means that the internet is not an option for support.

Whatever someone's age, a diagnosis of dementia is likely to come as a body blow. We, therefore, ask that you regard the stories that follow as pathways to understanding the realities of that disruption, even for older people. Think of each story as a 'teacher' if you will – that is, of having the capacity to hold your attention and inform you about the topic (Frank, 2010). We hope that you not only engage with each story carefully, but also reflect critically on your responses to the chain of care events contained within them. In particular, consider the extent to which each story sparks within you a new way of seeing a situation. This is because 'stories work with people, for people, and always stories work *on* people, affecting what people are able to see as real, as possible, and as worth doing or best avoided' (Frank, 2010: 3). We will guide you as to the point of each story and highlight what we think each story is doing, but ultimately the value of the story will be down to you and your imagination and questions.

The following real-life stories have been carefully selected to illustrate various points about relationality, care and citizenships in the context of people with a dementia living at home. At the heart of each story is recognition and respect for the person with a dementia. The first two stories, (1) William and (2) Bridget, are based on information we have sought and gathered from people within our own social networks. Hence, identifying details, such as names and place of residence, have been changed to protect their identity. The next two stories – (3) Masami Hayata, caring for his mother and young son and (4) Malcolm and Nigel – are told using material we have found in public sources. Together we hope that these stories will provide an understanding of not only the disruptive nature of dementia, but also more critically, how recognition and respect for the person living with a dementia, and the relationships they are in, can create new futures.

1 William

This first story is about William, an 82-year-old widower with complex health care needs and a history of repeated avoidable hospital admissions who returns home with a paid live-in carer. William has osteoarthritis and has been confined to a wheelchair for some years. Before his wife died several attempts were made to persuade William to have social services come into the home to provide regular support, but William always politely refused, insisting it was not necessary. After his wife died, William adjusted to living on his own with the help of his daughters, who would phone and visit as often as they could. However, being confined to a wheelchair became problematic for William, as he would fall asleep in it for long periods, which in turn, led to two admissions to hospital for cellulitis. The situation prompted a best interest decision meeting to be held, which was attended by William, his General Practitioner, Community Psychiatric Nurse (CPN) and two daughters. During this meeting, the GP succeeded in persuading William that there was a problem but he was unable to realise it, after which home carers started to visit William four times a day to provide regular care and support. This arrangement worked quite well for a few months. Unfortunately, the home carers would finish at nine in the evening, which was too early for William to go to bed, and so he spent the nights in a wheelchair, resulting once again in an admission to hospital for cellulitis.

The provision of quality home care is an essential component of supporting people with a dementia to remain at home and a major area of spending for local authorities (Alzheimer's Society, 2011). People with a dementia living alone are more likely to receive home care in their own homes (Miranda-Castillo, Woods, & Orrell, 2010). However, the care provided is often task orientated and problems often arise from the inconsistency of home care workers and timings, which can be unhelpful to people with a dementia (Alzheimer's Society, 2011). The problem is homecare workers are not adequately trained or remunerated to deal with the range of challenges they encounter, notably a lack of time to engage with clients and talk to them about their care needs – as one report says, 'we expect a lot of home care workers' (Koehler, 2014: ii).

For William in hospital, a diagnosis of a dementia had been made and he was deemed to lack the capacity to make a decision about his long-term care. As a result, the CPN started looking for a live-in carer as soon as William was admitted to hospital. The CPN knew that legally all available options had to be trialled before residential care was considered. Family members had asked that the live-in carer was male and could speak English. The care agency found a middle-aged man from Eastern Europe; his English was not fluent, but his manner was calm, gentle and quiet. Much to the surprise of family members, William readily accepted the live-in carer into his home. The two men built a convivial relationship; the carer was gentle, kind and quiet, and William seemed to enjoy the time they spent together. Moreover, William's physical and mental health improved; he was drinking and eating properly and had constant companionship. One of the unexpected bonuses of having a live-in carer was that he could hear and answer the telephone for William who was hard of hearing. Before the arrangement, one family member would ring every evening, but William either did not hear it or he mistook the TV remote control for the telephone handset, so they did not get a response. Afterwards, when the phone rang, the live-in carer would answer and pass the phone to William. As a result, the family believed, William's sense of the 'here and now' improved and he was less forgetful.

The story of William decentres the spousal 'care' relationship and opens up new possibilities and expectations for home care. It shows how it is worth trying new arrangements, even when family members think they may not work and they are not the cultural norm. The more traditional script, certainly in the UK, is for an older person to move into a care home when their health care needs are this complex, and they have been admitted to hospital several times. A refreshingly different care script is forged through this story, one in which the law is respected and the person with a dementia takes centre stage; thus, an alternative care package is set up. In particular, the story shows what it means to respect a person's right to live in the community. However, the story also raises important questions about the ethics of employing migrant care workers who may have care and citizenship concerns of their own.

Currently, in an increasing number of countries and cultures, including India, the USA and Singapore as well as the UK, live-in carers offer a practical solution for individuals and families in need of day and night care. Some families may prefer and be in a financial position to employ a person to provide round the clock support, so the person with a dementia can stay at home. For example, in a review of carers' accounts of arranging palliative care for their relatives with a dementia, the researchers found several incidences of a live-in carer being employed (Raymond et al., 2014). Whilst live-in care is a valued option for many individual households, the arrangement needs to be seen within a global socio-political context – e.g. employing foreign domestic workers shifts the responsibilities of care away from nation states (Yeoh & Huang, 2010). Only time will tell whether live-in carers become a long-term care option for more people in the future.

2 Bridget

The next story is about respectful relational care, with a visiting home care worker. It involves a woman named Bridget who lived on her own in Ireland following the death of her husband. Bridget's family lived in Australia and were involved in her care through weekly or more frequent phone conversations and regular visits. The story tells of how ordinary life changes and is disrupted when you live on your own with an undiagnosed dementia.

In many countries, older women are more likely to live alone, particularly due to the death of a partner. In the UK, for example, 22% of women aged 65–74 are widowed compared to 9% of men of the same age (Alzheimer's Research UK, 2015). For Bridget, in the years after becoming widowed her world got smaller as her health declined. Her short-term memory was degraded but still functioned adequately well. She could be paranoid and argumentative but was still able to retain good relationships with a close group of friends. Her mental agility and concentration were poor, restricting her ability to engage in fast-moving conversations with more than two people. She was unable to interpret written articles, official correspondence or radio/tv news. This was interpreted by her GP as being down to a series of mini-strokes rather than dementia. She did engage in one-on-one conversations on repetitive topics. Her physical condition deteriorated, primarily due to weight loss from not eating, to a point where her abilities to walk and get in and out of bed were restricted. Her weight loss was due to poor appetite rather than forgetting to eat.

As Bridget got weaker and lost the ability to walk anything more than short distances, her physical world contracted from her neighbourhood, to her house, finally to the ground floor of her home. Her circle of friends contracted down to about five regular visitors. Her interest in the world contracted to a handful of repetitive topics. Her diet contracted from one of adequate nutrition and balance to one consisting of primarily bread and porridge.

For five years, Bridget received a home help service provided by the state health service. Bernadette, an experienced home help provider, was assigned to visit Bridget five days a week. However, unlike other stories of people living at home in receipt of home help, Bernadette remained Bridget's carer for the remainder of Bridget's time living at home. While Bridget was uneasy and somewhat paranoid about accepting help initially, Bernadette won her over with kindness and persistence. They eventually formed a very close relationship that was the most crucial single factor in Bridget being able to achieve her goal of being able to live at home for as long as she did. The relationship worked because:

- The relationship was given time to develop. Bernadette remained Bridget's primary carer for five years. This consistency was fundamental to building the relationship.
- Bernadette committed to building a relationship with Bridget. She used her experience and personality to overcome Bridget's initial mistrust. In time the relationship grew into a true friendship
- Overcoming day-to-day challenges required experience, persistence and kindness. Bernadette exhibited all these characteristics and was truly dedicated to her job.

Bernadette determined what Bridget needed and tailored her role to those needs. For instance: she ensured that food was available and frequently prepared basic meals and sat with Bridget while she ate; she ensured that medicines were collected and consumed and encouraged Bridget to go for brief walks with her, to the best of Bridget's ability; she ensured that Bridget maintained basic personal hygiene. Bernadette had the time and desire to build strong relationships and was committed to providing the best support possible. To put it simply, she cared.

Other community service options were offered to Bridget but were less successful. This included, for example:

- Meals on wheels was provided to Bridget but her poor appetite and her paranoid concerns about the quality of the food meant she rarely ate it. She was more likely to eat with Bernadette's encouragement.
- A personal alarm was installed in the house, but Bridget refused to wear the pendant, as she could not be convinced that it was of value.
- Weekend home help was offered through a private service provider. This failed because different home help people were assigned each day. This lack of consistency meant there was no time for Bridget to overcome her distrust of strangers and to build relationships with them. The home help people assigned to her tended to be younger and less experienced in dealing with older people with complex needs. They also tended to be from overseas and Bridget found their accents very difficult to understand.

Bridget's primary medical support was provided by her GP and occasional visits by a community nurse. Care was focused on her physical condition, primarily monitoring a long-standing cardiac condition and providing a hip replacement. Her mental condition was not closely observed, perhaps because it did not exhibit all symptoms of dementia and because the decline was slow and prolonged. Her deteriorating mental condition was attributed to a series of mini-strokes. Bridget died in the summer of 2012 aged 88 years, following three months in a local general hospital. She was formally diagnosed with a dementia during this period in hospital, and end-stage dementia was determined as the cause of death and recorded on her death certificate.

Bridget's story shows what is possible when home care services provide relationship care. The benefits of a relationship-centred approach to people with a dementia have long been recognised (see, for example, Nolan, Ryan, Enderby, & Reid, 2002). However, much of this work has focused on care home settings (e.g. Rockwell, 2008) or family relationships (Nolan et al., 2002), rather than the relationships people with a dementia have with home care workers. Yet, as this story indicates, getting this relationship right can make all the difference to whether someone is able to enjoy a liveable life at home. Furthermore, it is a model of positive practice that home care providers can and do offer. For example, 'The Raglan Project' is an at-home care service that supports 14 people living with a dementia in a small rural community in Wales (Spencer, 2014). The model of service is relationship centred and critically, 'staff are given autonomy to support the choices of the service user, balancing physical needs with social and emotional needs, and taking the time to get to know the person' (p. 29). This has to be the way forward for home care services.

3 Masami Hayata: Caring for his mother and young son

The next story involves a relationship between three people: Masami Hayata, an ad executive, his young son and ailing mother – all of whom share a home in Japan. Although it is not explicitly stated, Masami's mother most likely has advanced dementia, as she is in her late 80s and completely dependent on others to meet her care needs. Globally, it is estimated that 13% of people aged 60 years and over are dependent (i.e. in need of frequent help or care beyond that habitually required by a healthy adult) – just over half of whom will have a dementia (Prince, Prina, & Guerchet, 2013). Women aged 65 years are more likely to be dependent in later life than men are. This particular story is compelling as it shows how it is possible for a highly dependent older person with a dementia to live with dignity at home, with her adult child and grandson.

The story is told in a short documentary film shot in Tokyo, called *Taller Than the Trees* (director Megan Mylan), which at the time of writing is available to view on Vimeo. The film is around 15 minutes long and shows Masami caring for his mother, who is completely dependent on him (and paid carers who we do not see) to meet her needs. The film is shot when Masami Hayata's wife is away from home working, and so he is caring for both his mother and their young son, whilst also going out to work himself. Globally, two-thirds of primary dementia caregivers are female, rising to more than 70% in lower-middle-income countries (Coreld, 2017: 3). Thus, a male caregiver is atypical, and perhaps more of a 'story' to the filmmaker.

There are several poignant scenes and interchanges in this film, which are relevant to our discussion of diversity and care and citizenship at home. One is when the son says of his mother as she lies in bed, not apparently doing very much, 'she is working hard through this phase (of her life)'. This is significant because it seems to give this woman agency, which is assumed to be lacking in the advanced phases of dementia. Furthermore, it serves to dignify her dependency, as it suggests that she is, in fact, ageing (or even dying?) well. Another striking scene in the film is when Masami Hayata is on a radio programme being interviewed about how he manages his work and caring responsibilities; he is asked, 'Why do you not give up work (to care for your mother full-time)?'. In the UK, the question would more likely be, 'Why do you not place her in a care home?'.

The story of Masami Hayata caring for his mother exemplifies the East Asian notion of filial piety – an important virtue and primary duty of respect, obedience and care for one's parent and elderly family members. Thus, as one cultural gerontologist points out, 'in countries throughout Asia and in most of the developing world, living intimately with others in a condition of appropriate inter/dependence is generally regarded as much more normal and valued than living independently' (Lamb, 2015: 38). Meaning that advancing care and citizenship at home is culturally situated and subject to regional variations.

One significant omission from this film is an insight into the informal/formal carer nexus. As already mentioned, paid carers visit Masami's mother, but we do not see them in the film. The only reference made to paid care staff (and how the viewer knows that they visit) is when Masami Hayata returns home after work one day to find his mother lying in wet clothing and bedding and says to her 'I'm sorry they left you like this', at which point he takes her to the bathroom, and in our view, bathes her in a completely dignified way. For example, at one point we hear the young son walking towards the bathroom as he wants to talk to his father, but his father asks him to wait outside as his mother is still naked. Bartlett has shown the film *Taller Than the Trees* to nursing students, one of whom perceived the bathing scene as an invasion of the mother's privacy and felt that it would be preferable for a formal care worker to carry out this activity (rather than her son). While this is an understandable perspective, it is rooted in a Westernised ideal of care and ageing. As we have already outlined, values such as privacy vary across cultures.

4 Malcolm and Nigel

This final story is about a gay couple – Malcolm (who has vascular dementia) and his partner Nigel, both of whom are in their 80s. The story is taken directly from a Guidance document for managers and leaders on *Dementia and Diversity*

(Skills for Care, 2014: 13). We have selected it to explore further the relational elements of care at home, and in particular, the advocacy role of care partners, including dementia advisors.

BOX 2.3 THE STORY OF MALCOLM AND NIGEL

Malcolm is 83 and has vascular dementia. He has difficulties with speech and swallowing. Malcolm also has expressive communication difficulties and is unable to coordinate his movements to write or point to pictures. Not being able to find the words he needs has been extremely distressing for him. Malcolm is highly educated, having gone to grammar school and then university before becoming a political journalist, travelling all over the world. Malcolm met Nigel at university, where they both studied politics, and have lived together as partners since 1956. They have continued to describe themselves as friends due to the discrimination they witnessed gay friends experiencing at that time.

Over the past year, Malcolm has experienced increased difficulty swallowing and almost continual chest infections. In addition, he is no longer able to bear weight. Malcolm receives private home care visits three times a day; usually from a care worker called Moira, with whom Nigel is very close. Malcolm's GP, who is also a family friend, is very supportive and they receive regular visits from the Alzheimer's Society dementia advisor – Celia.

Nigel is caring and constantly with Malcolm. However, in his grief Nigel has become increasingly distressed and angry, blaming Malcolm's lifestyle for his illness as Malcolm used to enjoy smoking, malt whisky and long afternoons in the pub. Malcolm and Nigel's partnership has not been formalised and there is no lasting power of attorney. This can be frustrating for Nigel as he feels his opinions are not listened to and that he is not being included in decisions about Malcolm's care and support, even though he often has helpful suggestions about Malcolm's preferences from their life together.

One day when Nigel was feeling particularly frustrated he spoke to Celia and told her how he had been feeling. Celia told Nigel to also speak to their friend, Malcolm's GP, and she would look into arranging additional support. A Mental Capacity Act Best Interest Meeting was set up between Nigel, Moira and her supervisor, Malcolm's GP and a social worker where they decided to provide palliative support but discontinue the current course of antibiotics, which had become ineffective in treating Malcolm's repeated chest infections.

Nigel is now very involved in Malcolm's care planning. He's involved Malcolm in reminiscence work, looking through some of the old papers that Malcolm used to work on. This has encouraged Malcolm to use some of the articles to help him find words to communicate his preferences. Nigel now feels much more involved and supported. He and Malcolm are getting on well and Malcolm is spending more time out of bed during the day, with the help of a hoist provided to help him get out of bed. Malcolm and Nigel's story shows the importance of involving a partner in care planning and also the role the mental capacity act can play even when the partnership has not been formalised, as is often the case in LGBT relationships, particularly for those of an older generation.

Taken directly from Skills for Care (2016: 13)

Malcolm and Nigel's story shows what is possible when people tell other people what they need and how they feel. Having to effectively 'come out' about one's sexuality to service providers is something that other people in a gay or lesbian relationship have had to do (Price, 2010). Fortunately, in Nigel's case, the response was a constructive one, as it created the opportunity for a best interest's meeting in which both he and the Dementia Advisor played a vital role. Thereafter, the relationship between these two men improved, as Nigel seemed more able to show he cared for and about Malcolm, and Malcolm himself enjoyed more freedoms (i.e. getting out of bed and talking more).

Gender has been a neglected dimension in public discourse related to people with a dementia. Those living with this condition have been portrayed in policies and strategies in gender-neutral terms as 'people with dementia' and 'family carers' as if gender does not matter when clearly it does. The discourse is beginning to change, as evidenced by the growing number of reports related to women and dementia (see, for example, Erol, Brooker, & Peel, 2015). However, as one of us has argued elsewhere, 'gender does not equal women: men are at risk of oppression too, but not from being a man' (Bartlett, Gjernes, Lotherington, & Obstefelder, 2016: 11). The studies we reviewed for this scoping review showed how 'one social identity could intersect with another to create disadvantage' (p. 12). Therefore, going back to Malcolm and Nigel, both of these men were at risk of marginalisation because they were in a gay relationship. Malcolm had the further potential disadvantage of a dementia diagnosis. However, in their favour, they were both highly educated, and Nigel had the resources to advocate for both himself and Malcolm. All these factors intersect and matter when seeking to understand life at home for citizens with a dementia and their family carers.

Closing comments

According to care geographers, it is important to 'reimagine care as not just relational but also as a resource flow' (Atkinson, Lawson, & Wiles, 2011: 569). This means thinking about how and where care is sourced and resourced. While there are obviously differences between the stories told in this chapter, there are similarities and connections too. The main unifier being that the displaying of dementia symptoms brings with it new relational struggles and currents.

For William and Bridget, these centred around making a new relationship, with someone from outside the family, work; in both cases, their health and well-being was contingent upon this relationship and the provision of respectful care by a home care worker. In contrast, Masami Hayata and his mother were relating to each other in a way that they would not have done before the illness – that is, in a more embodied and material way (bathing, changing bedsheets, moving in and out of a wheelchair). Both parties would have felt the emotional and physical demands of such a relationship. Similarly, the relational dynamics between Malcolm and Nigel had obviously changed and were continuing to change, as both men adjusted to their caring roles and responsibilities with the support of others who cared about them. This shows how fundamentally, advancing care and citizenship at home is about recognition and respect for the person living with a dementia, and the relationships and spaces in which they reside.

As this chapter on citizenships has shown, there is a value to storytelling for understanding life at home for people with a dementia. There are many other stories that could be told and that should be told. We have selected those which we think best mobilises the idea of care and citizenship at home. Our response to these stories may, of course, be different from yours. You may not, for example, have responded to the film *Taller Than the Trees* in the same way as we have done. Nevertheless, we hope that by sharing these stories the relational element of peoples' lives is foregrounded, and the struggles that individuals and families living with a dementia face, around the world, are better understood. Finally, it has been our intention in this opening chapter to introduce the core ideas and values that underpin this book, namely, social citizenship and the ethics of care.

References

Alzheimer's Research UK. (2015). Women and dementia: A marginalised majority. Cambridge: Alzheimer's Research UK, 1–13.

Alzheimer's Society. (2011). *Support. Stay. Save.* https://www.alzheimers.org.uk/download/downloads/id/1030/support_stay_save.pdf

Atkinson, S., Lawson, V., & Wiles, J. (2011). Care of the body: Spaces of practice. *Social & Cultural Geography, 12*(6), 37–41. https://doi.org/10.1080/14649365.2011.601238

Bartlett, R. (2007). 'You can get in alright but you can't get out': Social exclusion and men with dementia in nursing homes: Insights from a single case study. *Quality in Ageing and Older Adults, 8*(2), 16–26. https://doi.org/10.1108/14717794200700009

Bartlett, R. (2014). Citizenship in action: The lived experiences of citizens with dementia who campaign for social change. *Disability & Society, 29*(8), 1291–1304. https://doi.org/10.1080/09687599.2014.924905

Bartlett, R., Gjernes, T., Lotherington, A.-T., & Obstefelder, A. (2016). Gender, citizenship and dementia care: A scoping review of studies to inform policy and future research. *Health & Social Care in the Community, 26*(1), 14–26. https://doi.org/10.1111/hsc.12340

Bryden, C. (2005). *Dancing with Dementia: My Story of Living Positively with Dementia.* London: Jessica Kingsley Publishers.

Bury, M. (1982). Chronic illness as biographical disruption. *Sociology of Health and Illness, 4*(2), 167–182. http://onlinelibrary.wiley.com/doi/10.1111/1467-9566.ep11339939/full

Coreld, S. (2017). Women and Dementia A Global Challenge. *Global Alzheimer's & Dementia Action Alliance*. https://www.gadaalliance.org/wp-content/uploads/2017/02/Women-Dementia-A-Global-Challenge_GADAA.pdf

Erol, R., Brooker, D., & Peel, E. (2015). Women and dementia: A global research review. London: Alzheimer's Disease International.

ERSO. (2014). A good life with dementia. London: Red & Yellow Care

Frank, A. (1994) Just listening: Narrative and deep illness. *Family Systems and Health, 16*(3), 197–212.

Frank, A. (2010) *Letting Stories Breathe: A Socio-narratology.* Chicago: The University of Chicago Press.

Hansen, T. B. (2015). Citizenship as horizon. *Citizenship Studies, 19*(2), 229–232. https://doi.org/10.1080/13621025.2015.1005953

Hulko, W. (2009). From 'not a big deal' to 'hellish': Experiences of older people with dementia. *Journal of Aging Studies, 23*(3), 131–144. https://doi.org/10.1016/j.jaging.2007.11.002

Hayes, J., Zimmerman, M. K., & Boylstein, C. (2010). Responding to symptoms of Alzheimer's disease: Husbands, wives, and the gendered dynamics of recognition and disclosure. *Qualitative Health Research, 20*(8), 1101–1115. http://journals.sagepub.com/doi/abs/10.1177/1049732310369559

Kerpershoek, L., de Vugt, M., Wolfs, C., Jelley, H., Orrel, M., Woods, B., … Verhey, F. (2016). Access to timely formal dementia care in Europe: Protocol of the Actifcare (ACcess to Timely Formal Care) study. *BMC Health Services Research, 16*(1), 423. https://doi.org/10.1186/s12913-016-1672-3

Koehler, I. (2014). Key to care: Report of the Burstow Commission on the future of the home care workforce (December). London: The Local Democracy Think Tank.

Lamb, S. (2015). Beyond the view of the West: Ageing and anthropology. In J. Twigg & W. Martin (Eds.), *Routledge Handbook of Cultural Gerontology* (pp. 37–45). London: Routledge.

Maratou-Alipranti, M., & Tastsoglou, E. (2010). Rethinking citizenship with women in focus. In Abraham, M., Ngan-ling, C., Maratou-Alipranti, L., & Tastsoglou, E. (Eds.), *Contours of Citizenship. Women, Diversity and Practices of Citizenship* (1st ed., pp. 1–21). Surrey, UK: Ashgate Publishing.

Miranda-Castillo, C., Woods, B., & Orrell, M. (2010). People with dementia living alone: What are their needs and what kind of support are they receiving? *International Psychogeriatrics, 22*(4), 607–617. https://doi.org/10.1017/S104161021000013X

Mitchell, W. (2018). *Somebody I Used to Know.* London: Bloomsbury.

Nolan, M., Ryan, T., Enderby, P., & Reid, D. (2002). Towards a more inclusive vision of dementia care practice and research. *Dementia, 1*(2), 193–211. https://doi.org/10.1177/147130120200100206

O'Connor, D., Phinney, A., & Hulko, W. (2010). Dementia at the intersections: A unique case study exploring social location. *Journal of Aging Studies, 24*(1), 30–39. https://doi.org/10.1016/j.jaging.2008.08.001

Pitt, E. (2017). *Kate Swaffer: Activist, Academic.* http://stand.uow.edu.au/kate-swaffer-activist-academic/

Price, E. (2010). Coming out to care: Gay and lesbian carers' experiences of dementia services. *Health & Social Care in the Community, 18*(2), 160–168. https://doi.org/doi:10.1111/j.1365-2524.2009.00884.x

Prince, M., Prina, M., & Guerchet, M. (2013). World Alzheimer report 2013 journey of caring: An analysis of long-term care for dementia (September). London: Alzheimer's Disease International.

Raymond, M., Warner, A., Davies, N., Iliffe, S., Manthorpe, J., & Ahmedzhai, S. (2014). Palliative care services for people with dementia: A synthesis of the literature reporting the views and experiences of professionals and family carers. *Dementia*, *13*(1), 96–110. https://doi.org/10.1177/1471301212450538

Rockwell, J. (2008). *Relationships as remedy: Meeting the social and emotional needs of elders living in residential care*. MA Thesis. University of British Columbia.

Sandberg, L. J. (2018). Dementia and the gender trouble?: Theorising dementia, gendered subjectivity and embodiment. *Journal of Aging Studies* (in press), 0–1. https://doi.org/10.1016/j.jaging.2018.01.004

Shippee, N. D., Shah, N. D., May, C. R., Mair, F. S., & Montori, V. M. (2012). Cumulative complexity: A functional, patient-centered model of patient complexity can improve research and practice. *Journal of Clinical Epidemiology*, *65*(10), 1041–1051. https://doi.org/10.1016/j.jclinepi.2012.05.005

Spencer, E. (2014). Models of positive practice to support people with dementia and their carers in Wales, with a primary focus on North Wales (August). Denbighshire, Wales: *Denbighshire County Council*, 1–78.

Swaffer, K. (2016). *What the Hell Happened to My Brain? Living Beyond Dementia*. London: Jessica Kingsley Publishers.

Yeoh, B. S. A., & Huang, S. (2010). Foreign domestic workers and home-based care for elders in Singapore. *Journal of Aging & Social Policy*, *22*(1), 69–88. https://doi.org/10.1080/08959420903385635

3

ENABLING LIFE AT HOME

Introduction

The aim of this chapter is to provide a detailed review of the progress and prospects for enabling people with a dementia to live well at home. Enabling is a term often used in disability studies to draw attention to the practical implications of living with an impairment and the societal barriers that many people with a disability face. In a key text written by disability scholars over 20 years ago, the vision was for an 'enabling society' where there are no restrictions on lifestyle and people with a disability feel able to ask for help (Hales, 1996). Since then scholars have explored the topic of disability extensively, and sought to make this utopia a reality for the millions of people living with a disability worldwide. However, very little attention has been paid in this scholarship to those with a progressive cognitive impairment or older people with disabilities generally. This is unfortunate as much of the work is relevant when it comes to thinking about enabling people with a dementia to live well at home.

Our aim here is to draw on this scholarship and focus on enabling people with a dementia to live at home. Enabling people with disabilities to participate in society as equal citizens is a long-standing theme within disability studies (e.g. Hales, 1996). Similarly, the aim of this chapter is to provide a thoughtful account of what is known about enabling people with a dementia to live at home. The hope is that discussion will stimulate thinking about what might be possible for people with a dementia (and their carers) who live at home. The vocabulary of enablers, enabling and enablement is used to promote a constructive understanding of making life at home liveable for people with a dementia. The chapter draws on empirical research in order to conceptualise enabling care and citizenship and to show what works. Our intention is not to shy away from the more challenging aspects of life at home for people with a dementia but to foreground what is possible. Moreover, we do not mean to exclude care homes, but to ensure that individuals with a dementia have a meaningful choice as to where they live.

At the centre of the discussion are people living with a dementia and the societal structures, cultural norms and environmental demands that surround us. We are thinking here of constructs like gender, sexuality and ethnicity; normative ideals like marriage, having children and grandchildren; and everyday stresses such as using busy roads and public transport systems. There has been a tendency in dementia studies to focus solely on 'the dementia' in isolation of other matters and to centralise the needs of 'caregivers'. Our intention in this chapter is to review and discuss relevant evidence from the perspective of people with a dementia and in the broader context of the multiple environments in which that person lives. As one campaign group notes,

> the quality of life for all citizens, but especially for the growing number of older citizens and those living with chronic conditions is determined mainly by how far the physical and social environment of their daily lives supports autonomy, independent living, social connectivity and meaningful social participation.
>
> *(Agile Ageing Alliance:9)*

Thus, we consider how the environment, not just the caregiver, supports and enables an individual with a dementia to live at home.

Enabling support systems for people with a dementia

The chapter is organised around an idea from disability studies of enabling support systems, in which the 'interface between individuals and the environments' is paramount (Litvak & Enders, 2001: 711). We have taken the idea and adapted it to frame our discussion of enabling people with a dementia to live well at home. There are four key components or enablers of such a system, all of which take the perspective of the person with dementia. These are (1) relational ('*who* do you need in your life?'), (2) service-level ('*what* do want from formal services, and *when* do you want it?'), (3) environmental (*where* do you feel happy and in control?) and (4) structural ('*how* can legislators create the right environment?'). The elements overlap but are discussed separately to tease out and highlight the essential features of an enabling support system. Even though the idea may seem like a static singular explanation, 'support systems, whatever their configuration, are intensely and intimately individual; they are also dynamic' (Litvak & Enders, 2001: 711). This means they can and need to change as and when a person's situation changes. Thus, throughout this chapter, we use the idea of enabling support systems to frame and provoke discussion about making life at home liveable for people with a dementia.

Like the disability scholars who advocate for an enabling support system, we are interested in the role of supports in improving 'functional ability' at home and whilst out and about in the community (Litvak & Enders, 2001: 711). Functional ability is about being able to 'perform fundamental physical and mental actions used in daily life, such as mobilising, seeing, hearing, remembering and speaking' (Verbrugge & Jette, 1994). Basic human tasks like these are essential for participating in domestic and community activities. However, having a dementia can make them incredibly difficult to carry out. Sometimes this is due to the effects of the dementia, but more often than not it is because others start to 'take over' or treat the person with a dementia as completely incompetent. For example, researchers who have studied decision-making amongst couples affected by a dementia, have found that family members will dominate the conversation and make choices on the person's behalf (see, for example, Smebye, Kirkevold, & Engedal, 2012; Boyle, 2014). Others report that people with a dementia have found themselves living in a care home without having been afforded the chance to explore other options or decide for themselves whether that is where they want to live (Lord, Livingston, Robertson, & Cooper, 2016). Hence, in this chapter, we equate enabling life at home with promoting the functional abilities of people with a dementia to carry out their daily lives and participate as citizens.

Dementia is a disability that profoundly affects a person's ability to remember, so much so that one person described his experience of this disablement to Bartlett as 'the terror of forgetting'. Thus, enabling a person to function with a severely impaired memory is an area where most support is required (and where most research has focused). However, dementia can be more than memory; it creates sensory challenges such as 'brain blindness' where the brain is unable to process what it sees and hears properly (Houston, 2016). The novelist Terry Pratchett (1948–2015), who was diagnosed with Posterior Cortical Atrophy (PCA) – a rare form of Alzheimer's disease – initially visited an optometrist because he thought he had problems with his eyesight as he kept trying to put his coat on upside down. It is noteworthy that certain forms of dementia (such as PCA, Pick's disease and frontal-temporal lobe dementia) affect certain parts of the brain and so support may be needed in quite particular areas of daily functioning such as language and vision.

Dementia is often described as a *hidden* disability, as it is not always obvious to others that someone is cognitively impaired. This is how many of those who are dementia activists and still actively campaigning for social change often describe the condition. However, as the dementia progresses it can affect a person's facial expression, posture, gait and general ability to move around and complete routine manual tasks (like opening doors and eating) at which point the disability does become visible. The discernibility and fluctuating nature of dementias are important to note, as it means a person's ability to carry out everyday actions are likely to change over time and can shift dramatically depending on the environment in which they are in (Litvak & Enders, 2001).

According to disability scholars, 'disability is not a personal characteristic, but is instead a gap between personal capability and environmental demand' (Verbrugge & Jette, 1994: 1). For a person with a dementia, the gap is likely to be produced by not only the dementia but also other age-related conditions. In fact, it has been estimated that 95% of people with a dementia will also have at least one other long-term health condition or disability, such as diabetes, sight loss or stroke (Sube Banerjee, 2015), making dementia a particularly complex disability. For example, 'people with a pre-existing diagnosis of diabetes who are subsequently diagnosed with dementia may find their "hypo" awareness is comprised as their cognitive function deteriorates' (Sinclair et al., 2014: 11). Indeed, one of the respondents in a qualitative study conducted by Wilson (2012), who lived alone reported being admitted to hospital because she had no one to remind her to check her blood glucose or take insulin. Thus, to explore the subject of enabling life at home more fully, we need to consider not only the effects of dementia on functional ability but also how other impairments and health conditions can influence and destabilise a person's situation, as shown in Figure 3.1.

As well as equating enabling life at home with promoting functional abilities, we link it to stability. Acknowledging the conceptual work currently underway in Germany, which seeks to define and assess the stability of care arrangements at home for people with a dementia, we too consider stability as a significant enabler (see von Kutzleben, Reuther, Dortmann, & Holle, 2016 for more details of this work). Stability – keeping things constant and regular – is important because it can provide strength and support citizenship. As we explain in this chapter, it does this by helping to ensure that the person with a dementia has the tools and resources they require to do the everyday things they enjoy doing and have control over their lives. Therefore, in the discussion that follows, we regard

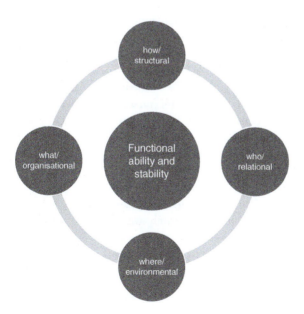

FIGURE 3.1 Elements of an enabling support system

stability as a central outcome for people with a dementia who live at home and those who support them.

The chapter begins by looking at the main reasons why people move into a care home before reviewing what we know about enabling people with a dementia to function at home. We begin with a discussion about the reasons why people move into a care home as this can reveal what individuals and families require from an enabling support system.

The reasons why people move into a care home

We know a lot about why people with a dementia move into a care home. There have been several major studies into this transition, which are important to note here as they reveal where support systems are weakest. One of the largest most recent studies looking at the transitions of care from private homes to long-term residential or nursing home care is the RightTimePlaceCare study, funded by the EU Health Framework. The study involved a consortium of multi-disciplinary researchers and clinicians from eight European countries, Estonia, Finland, France, Germany, Spain, Sweden, the Netherlands and the UK, and was completed between 2010 and 2013 (see Verbeek et al., 2012).

For the purposes of this book, we want to highlight the results from the Work Package, which looked at the transition phase from 'care at home', to 'care in a nursing home'. The work was based on a sample of 2014 dyads of people with a dementia and their informal caregivers; 1223 of whom lived at home and the person with a dementia was at risk of institutionalisation; the other 791 involved a person with a dementia who had recently moved into an institution. As explained in the summary available on the aforementioned website, 'the main questions were: why are these people being admitted to a nursing home, what is the quality of life of people with a dementia, what is the quality of care provided, and what is the burden for informal carers?' (p. 8). The team surveyed key stakeholders and found considerable variation between countries. For example, 'the severity of dementia can be an important reason for nursing home admission in one country, whereas in another country that is less important' (p. 8). However, one consistent factor associated with institutionalisation was found in all analyses (i.e. countries), and that was 'caregiver burden'. People with a dementia move into a care home because the person who is assisting them is no longer able to do so without seriously risking their own health and well-being.

A breakdown in carer support is a well-documented reason for why some people with a dementia move into a care home. Research over many years endorses the view that some of the effects of dementia are more troubling and challenging to deal with than others. These include incontinence, violent outbursts and leaving the house and getting lost, especially at night. For example, during her PhD study, Bartlett recalls talking to the husband of a woman with a dementia who he had just arranged to be moved into a care home because for him double incontinence was the 'final straw'. Other researchers have reported on how a nursing home placement was arranged for a man with a dementia following a critical incident in which 'he had angrily grasped his wife's wrists, demanding to know why she had made decisions about the day care centre without informing him. His wife used this incident to underline his need for being institutionalised' (Smebye et al., 2016: 8). Others have analysed the predictive factors for institutional care and drawn the conclusion that repeatedly getting lost may lead to institutionalisation (Banerjee et al., 2003). Finally, researchers have found that the 'desire to institutionalise' a person with a dementia may be stronger for male caregivers when the relationship with their wife *before* diagnosis was poor (Winter, Gitlin, & Dennis, 2011: 221). All of this highlights the weakness of a system that relies upon one person to provide assistance.

Another large-scale study conducted recently in Canada, called 'Seniors in Transition', also found that people with severe cognitive impairment moved into a care home because the caregiver was no longer able to continue supporting the person at home. However, it was not the main reason. The prime reason for a person moving into a care home was that the initial assessment had taken place in hospital rather than in the person's own home (CIHI, 2017: 20). As a member of the working group said:

> it is difficult for hospital staff to maintain a focus on helping seniors return to their normal living arrangements when hospitals are over capacity and under pressure to decrease length of stays of their patients ... (hence) seniors who could perhaps return home with assistance, are placed into residential care.
>
> *(p. 29)*

This is significant, as it highlights the time-space dimensions of care (Bowlby, 2012), and in particular, how someone can be transferred into a care home because of a perceived lack of time and space. Furthermore, it reinforces a point we made in Chapter two about the rarity of someone with a dementia returning home following admission to hospital.

We know that people who live alone are more likely to move into a care home, and these individuals are predominately women aged 85 years and over. At least two studies have calculated the odds for people who live alone of moving into a care home. One is the 'Seniors in Transition' study; it found that seniors who lived alone (without a primary caregiver in the home) were 2.0 times more likely to enter residential care than those who lived with their primary caregiver. The other is a longitudinal study of 100 people with a dementia; it found that having a co-resident carer made admission to a care home 20 times less likely over a one-year period (Banerjee et al., 2003). This would suggest that people with a dementia need some form of round-the-clock support as the condition worsens.

In summary, people with a dementia move into a care home because of a lack of appropriate support and assistance. Evidence is strongest about 'caregiver burden', but arguably this is because there have been caregiver burden scales for researchers to use since the 1980s. As understanding of how different organisational practices and living arrangements expands, the knowledge base will inevitably grow and diversify. Having reviewed the main reasons for moving into a care home, we now turn our attention to making it possible for people with a dementia to live at home. As already indicated, our intention is to present and explain the key elements of an enabling support system from the perspective of the person with a dementia. These are (1) relational ('*who* do you need in your life?'); (2) service-level ('*what* do want from formal services, and *when* do you want it?'); (3) environmental (*where* do you feel happy and in control?) and (4) structural ('*how* can legislators create the right environment?'). Although each of these enablers is discussed separately, they are inevitably interlinked.

Relational enablers

Relational enablers are about 'who' a person with a dementia needs to support their life at home and the interpersonal dynamics that unfold in the process. Arguably, this is *the* most important element of an enabling support system, as fundamentally enabling life at home is relational. It has been over 30 years since Tom Kitwood wrote his classic text: *Dementia Reconsidered: the person comes first*. Since then, research on social relations and relationship-centred care has grown enormously, especially in relation to care homes. Here, we are concerned with the domestic environment and, in particular, how relationships with people (and animals) can support functionality, stability and citizenship.

Citizenship has been defined as living successfully with others; it is a way of relational living in which the decisions and actions of one citizen must be understood in terms of their influence on the lives of others (Pols, 2017). Unfortunately, the onset of a dementia can disrupt the relationships and support strategies a person has nurtured during their life course. This may be due to 'a fear of exposure' and so people choose to distance themselves from activities in the community (Evans, Price, & Meyer, 2016: 11). Or a person with a dementia may feel embarrassed about their memory lapses and less interested in socialising and going out (Singleton, Mukadam, Livingston, & Sommerlad, 2017). Alternatively, it could be because others do not understand, or try to understand, what the person is going through. A recent systematic review of qualitative research related to the 'everyday interpersonal relationships, as experienced by people with a dementia' concluded that other people's responses are a critical factor in achieving social well-being (Patterson et al., 2017: 1).

Accounts of relational living by people with a dementia, demonstrate the capacity and determination of people to adapt. Furthermore, they show how relational encounters are valuable opportunities for promoting functionality and stability. In a systematic review of the research evidence on the experiences that people with a dementia have with others, researchers summarised the essence of the experience in terms of 'living a meaningful life in relational changes' (Eriksen et al., 2016: 342). The researchers critically reviewed 63 research articles published between January 2004 and May 2016, all of which made explicit the voices of people with a dementia and included descriptions of their experiences of lived relations with others. The majority of data were gathered from people with a dementia living at home. The points listed in Box 3.1 are all taken from the article and might be regarded in terms of relational enablers.

BOX 3.1 RELATIONAL ENABLERS

1. Understand *how* a person with dementia experiences the quality of a relationship, as this is more important than the number of social connections a person has.
2. Good quality relationships can be a buffer against anxiety and depression; poor quality ones can have the opposite effect.
3. People with dementia are likely to feel accepted and understood, by other people with dementia.
4. Recognise that some people with dementia will seek to protect themselves, either by maintaining social relationships or avoiding them.
5. Relationships with others can provide a sense of security and belonging; we feel like we mean something to other people and have particular tasks and roles.
6. People with dementia need to feel that they are still involved in their own life.

Eriksen et al. (2016: 342)

The extent to which a person with a dementia is able, or feels able, to maintain control over their life is an important relational enabler. Studies conducted in several countries have found this to be of paramount importance to people with a dementia. In fact, one of the earliest studies on community-based care for people with a dementia added 'lack of control' as an outcome measure once they had started interviewing participants with a dementia (Bamford & Bruce, 2005). Since then, several studies have sought to investigate how people with a dementia can be supported to achieve this. For example, an Australian study involving six individuals with a dementia (four women and two men) living in the community and aged between 54 and 78 years, found that individuals with a dementia value 'subtle support' – that is, knowing that support is available but it being available on their own terms (Featherstonehaugh, Tarzia, & Nay, 2013: 149). Elsewhere, Norwegian researchers spent time with ten people with moderate dementia to explore participation in decision-making (five persons were living at home and five had moved to sheltered housing or to a nursing home. The mean age was 83 years and only two were men). Although the team found varying degrees of ability to participate in decision-making, people responded positively to being 'positioned as capable of influencing decisions' (Smebye et al., 2012: 241).

Clearly, it is important to learn how men and women with a dementia would like to be supported as it may not be in the way those around them expect.

Other researchers have reported on the gendered nature of control. Being able to stay in control are very different experiences for men and women. For example, an interview study on intimacy conducted in the US, involving 13 men and 15 women whose spouses had a diagnosis of a dementia, found gendered responses to maintaining a love life. On the one hand, 'the status hierarchy was preserved for caregiver husbands, and this enabled them to continue intimate relations with impaired wives. The husband remained in control of the relationship and continued to initiate sexual intimacy' (Hayes, Boylstein, & Zimmerman, 2009: 57). On the other, they found that men with a dementia were positioned in a somewhat contemptuous way by their wives; for example, they were more likely to be described as 'baby like' by their spouses, and one participant spoke with incredulity as to how her husband could 'remember' how to have sex but not do other things around the home (p. 54). In another study looking at everyday decision-making between married couples when one partner has a dementia, it was found that 'gendered patterns of authority or control were apparent in the couples' decision-making dynamics, indicating that gender inequality in relationships persists even when women develop dementia' (Boyle, 2014: 336). This area of work suggests that traditional gender dynamics can affect whether or not someone with dementia is able, or feels able, to maintain control over their life.

Of course, not every person with a dementia is married and living with a spouse. Nevertheless, relational and gendered dynamics are still important to consider, as people with a dementia who live alone are likely to have some contact with relatives either all of the time or during the day or night. Evans, Price and Meyer (2016) conducted an exploratory study into what clinicians perceive to be the main challenges, encountered by people with a dementia who live alone in the community; they began by asking the 21 participants this broad question: 'What do you believe to be the major challenges to the well-being of people who have dementia and live alone?'. The researchers found that the challenges were wide-ranging as living alone could take various forms; most commonly, it meant living in the community as the sole occupant of a house or unit. However, they also found cases of people living alone during the day; for example, one woman lived with her son who went to work all day. She had access to the house and garden, but he locked the garden gate to maintain her safety (p. 4). Other cases included people living alone at night, living alone temporarily (e.g. while a family member went on holiday) or living alone unexpectedly (e.g. after a spouse has died and other family members do not recognise the extent of the person's cognitive decline). Curiously, the researchers had a category for 'alone together' to describe a situation where both husband and wife have a dementia and live in their own home together. Finally, the researchers suggest that people can live 'alone with someone else' – that is, when they live with someone but receive no meaningful support. Perhaps one of the most disturbing cases uncovered by this research is of a woman who lived at the back of her ex-husband's flat, which was cluttered and contained mice, rats and pigeons. The ex-husband lived at the front and controlled her access (p. 4). This work highlights the diversity of living arrangements for people with a dementia and shows how care and citizenship are interlinked.

People with a dementia will have dealings with other people besides their spouses or relatives. Such relationships are likely to include friends, neighbours possibly, as well as others who live close by, such as shop workers, baristas, tradespeople, faith leaders and community police officers – even strangers on the street. In the Safer Walking GPS Project, we observed during the course of walking interviews the value of daily interactions with local people and being able to approach a stranger to ask for help. When one considers the larger picture of whom a person with a dementia might know, a potentially wider support network becomes possible – a point we return to in Chapter six on sharing responsibilities.

As already indicated, relational enablers are about 'who' is in a person's life and that includes other people with a dementia. The friendships people with a dementia have with other people with a dementia are an important source of support and are described as 'peer support'. Researchers who interviewed over 100 people with a dementia about their relationships with others found that 'peer support had positive emotional and social impact that was rooted in identification with others, a commonality of experience and reciprocity of support' (Keyes, Clarke, & Wilkinson, 2014: 560). Similarly, in a review of the literature on the experience of relations in dementia, researchers identified several studies, which emphasised the aspect of being with others with a dementia, as an 'expression of equality, comfort or safety' (Eriksen et al., 2016: 365). The work suggests that peer relationships are inherently supportive because a person with a dementia does not 'need to be more, or perform more than they are capable of doing' (p. 365). It also provides further evidence of how critical friendships and peer relationships are for people with a disability, as individuals 'in the same boat' can help one other (Worth, 2013: 114).

As well as support from family and friends, and other people generally, animals can provide a source of support and stability to people with a dementia. Pets can offer comfort to people with a dementia, especially those who live alone or spend long periods of time at home alone. As a leading charity found in their survey of loneliness, 'pets provide the person with dementia with a purpose. For example, dogs will always need walking, and all animals need to be fed. One woman living alone, when asked how she spends her day, explained that looking after the cats can take up a lot of her time. Another person described her cat as her best friend. Several respondents to the survey said that their pet helps them to overcome feelings of loneliness. As one person said: "My puppy helps me feel less lonely"' (Alzheimer's Society, 2013: 42). As well as countering loneliness, a well-behaved dog can support a person with wayfinding when out. In the Safer Walking GPS Project, we encountered a number of people with a dementia living at home who relied on their dog to get them back home safely.

However, the practical help an animal can provide is usually very limited, unless it has been trained as a service animal.

Service animals, primarily dogs, are trained to assist people with their daily tasks (Litvak & Enders, 2001). The 'Dementia Dogs' programme, currently only available in certain parts of Scotland, is perhaps the best (and only) example of such a system specifically for people with a dementia. The programme aims to train and provide dogs to help people with a dementia. According to their website, 'dogs can help people with a dementia maintain their waking, sleeping and eating routine, remind them to take medication, improve confidence, keep them active and engaged with their local community, as well as providing a constant companion who will reassure when facing new and unfamiliar situations' (http://dementiadog.org/about/how-we-help/). The programme is popular amongst people with a dementia; it would be good to see it extended to other parts of the UK and across the world.

Service-level enablers

Service-level enablers are about 'what' people need and 'when' they need it. In resource-rich countries, community-based services exist to enable people with a dementia to live at home – these are mainly care services but can include housing with care schemes, holidays and respite services, advocacy services and legal advice. It is beyond the scope of this chapter to describe every single type of service available to people with a dementia as services available in one part of a country or the world may not be available in another. Besides, our concern here is with what people need to support functionality and stability rather than what is actually available. Nevertheless, certain services and studies are discussed to highlight what is meant by service-level enablers, including, for example, new research on meeting centres and live-in carers.

Before discussing service-level enablers in detail, let us take a moment to consider what people with a dementia need and have a right to expect in terms of needs. In a systematic review of qualitative research studies, involving a combined sample of 345 people with varying degrees and forms dementia, researchers identified four factors that make people either happy or sad. According to people with a dementia, four factors, and the experience of connectedness or disconnectedness within each factor, influenced the quality of life. These factors, and the terms that represent connectedness and disconnectedness, were relationships (together vs alone), agency in life today (purposeful vs aimless), wellness perspective (well vs ill), and sense of place (located vs unsettled) (O'Rourke, Duggleby, Fraser, & Jerke, 2015). These factors provide a useful summation of peoples' needs. As for what citizens with a dementia have a right to expect, it is 'to live the life they choose and to be included in their community' (Article, 19, Convention on the Rights of Persons with Disabilities). In supporting individuals with a dementia to realise this right, the nature of support is key.

A focus on service-level enablers is important because at least a quarter of people with a dementia currently admitted to a residential or nursing home could be more appropriately supported in their own homes if more enhanced community services existed. Researchers, clinicians and others are therefore working hard to develop new services and interventions to enable people with a dementia to stay at home. For example, in the United States researchers have designed a randomised control trial to assess whether a home-based intervention can improve functional independence for clients in receipt of the Connecticut Home Care Program for Elders. The intervention, called Care of Persons with Dementia in their Environments (COPE), consists of ten sessions with an Occupational Therapist over a four-month period, and one face-to-face meeting and one phone call from an Advanced Practice Nurse (Fortinsky et al., 2016). One of the inclusion criteria for the study is 'planning to admit client to a nursing home in six months' so the intervention clearly aims to benefit older people with complex care needs and delay or prevent institutionalisation.

Another trial study, which commenced in Belgium at the start of 2016, seeks to determine whether in-home respite care is an effective strategy in supporting informal caregivers of people with a dementia (Vandepitte, Van Den Noortgate, Putman, Verhaeghe, & Annemans, 2016). Unlike the Connecticut study, the outcome measures relate to the well-being of the spouse (rather than the person with a dementia). The desired outcomes are to reduce 'caregiver burden' and improve the quality of life of the caregiver. The intervention group consists of a caregiver/care recipient receiving an in-home respite program called 'Baluchonnage' – a service provided by Baluchon Alzheimer's Belgium and particular to this country (p. 2). Whilst it is encouraging to see an emphasis on providing round-the-clock support, making a distinction between 'caregiver' and 'care recipient' in the way this study does (and many others do) is problematic.

It is problematic because it assumes that a person is one or the other (a caregiver or care recipient) when we know from the geographies of care literature that individuals alternate between these positions all the time (Bowlby, McKie, Gregory, & MacPherson, 2010). Even people with advancing dementia have the capacity to show they care. Take, for example, the intergenerational work involving older people with a dementia in care homes and young children, where both groups show they care for each other through play and laughter (Mendes, 2015). Thus, an enabling service needs to recognise the capacity of an individual with a dementia to care (as well as be cared for) and focus on the benefits of the service to the person with a dementia (as well as the person who supports them).

Another service-level enabler is flexible care arrangements. An increasing number of families are employing someone to live in their home – take, for example, the story of William and his paid personal assistant in Chapter 2. In some countries (such as India and China), this has always happened either due to the stigma of institutional care (Brijnath, 2012) and/or because specialist institutional care is lacking (Wu, Gao, & Dong, 2016). In other countries (such as Sweden and Singapore) personal assistants (PAs) have become part of the service culture.

For example, in Sweden if a person is diagnosed with a dementia before the age of 65, they are entitled to a personal assistant. In Singapore, the employment of 'live-in foreign domestic workers as care workers for older people has become one of the most common de facto models of providing care' (Yeoh & Huang, 2010). We have already highlighted in Chapter two, how the employment of migrant workers raises ethical questions. Here, we want to suggest that PAs provide another option for people who live at home. As Hellström and Larsson (2017: 140) point out, 'the introduction of personal assistance represents a significant step towards full citizenship in many countries like the UK and Sweden in the sense that their opportunities to take control over their own life are significantly improved'.

Services are only enabling if they provide the support that people need at the time it is needed. Sometimes community-based services are set up for people with a dementia and attendance is poor. We know of memory cafes that have sprung up for people with a dementia but discontinue because people did not use them. One can only assume it is because either people do not know about them, or they do not need or want the service on offer. One study explored the care arrangements of 84 people with a dementia living at home in a provincial–rural area in Germany. The most frequently used formal services were home care nursing services (53.0%), day care (49.4%) and respite care (29.6%), whereas 15.5% did not use any type of formal support (von Kutzleben, Reuther, Dortmann, & Holle, 2016). In another study, involving 18 family carers living in rural Tasmania, researchers found evidence of 'careful gatekeeping by carers in terms of who, among potential support providers, is admitted to their world and how far they penetrate' (Orpin, Stirling, Hetherington, & Robinson, 2012: 191).

Access to information is key to enablement. People with a dementia and family carers need to understand what is happening to them and what support they can expect. For example, according to research conducted in Sweden involving interviews with 110 caregivers of people with a dementia, 'getting information about the condition and about available services, and having someone to talk to, were seen as very important by the highest proportion of caregivers' (Alwin, Öberg, & Krevers, 2010). Unfortunately, research suggests this is a weakness in the system. In another study conducted in Australia involving culturally diverse communities, researchers found that participants did not know about services; many of the 121 families involved in the study had no idea what was available. In Australia, for example, researchers surveyed 152 carers of people with a dementia and found that they did not use day care and respite services because they associated them with negative outcomes, even though they may never have used the service (Phillipson, Magee, & Jones, 2013). This work suggests that services could do more to recognise the information needs and heterogeneity of people with a dementia, particularly those from black and minority ethnic communities.

Recognition is a key feature of inclusive citizenship (Lister, 2007). Recognition of difference, and in particular, respecting that some people will find dealing with dementia more challenging than others will – perhaps due to cultural norms and/or socioeconomic differences. For example, in recent work involving migrants from the Middle East living in Sweden, researchers found that people did not access community services because of strong cultural values linked to filial piety (Antelius, 2017). Similarly, in the UK researchers have been raising awareness of the support needs of Black and Minority Ethnic Communities as many families are reluctant to ask for help (e.g. Moriarty, Sharif, & Robinson, 2011). According to one housing provider, there needs to be a 'radical shift towards a personalized and coordinated model of care and support ... and the important contribution made by families, friends and wider community support networks needs to be recognised' (National Housing Federation & HACT, 2015: 8). With recognition, we can begin to move towards integrated care.

Integrated care is a service-enabler. This is when care services are well co-ordinated and closely aligned to the needs of clients (Shaw, Rosen and Rumbold, 2011). One example of a community-based integrated care service for people with a dementia is the Geriant model, which is provided by a Dutch organisation in the northern part of Noord-Holland province. Geriant provides an integrated set of services that includes diagnostics, clinical case management and treatment (Glimmerveen & Nies, 2015). Case management starts as soon as possible post-diagnosis, which for some people may only involve a phone call once or twice a year. In other more complex cases, it may involve a social geriatrician or other health care specialist. Wherever possible, family members or informal caregivers are engaged as care partners, and their support needs are met through counselling or advice giving (p. 4). The service is commonly regarded as an 'exemplary practice for community-based dementia care services' in the Netherlands and is estimated to cost on average eight euros a day per person.

The Admiral Nursing service, available to some families in the UK, is similar to the Geriant model in that it only employs and trains nurses and aims to reduce 'caregiver burden'. An Admiral Nurse's role is to provide specialist care and co-ordinate support – critically, they are there for the caregiver, rather than the person with a dementia (Bunn, Goodman, Pinkney, & Drennan, 2016). Bunn and her colleagues conducted a systematic review of the evidence on specialist Admiral Nurses and found that while caregivers value the service, evidence is weak as to its impact on enabling people with a dementia to live at home. Furthermore, we would suggest that it comes too late in a family's journey. As the authors point out though, the service does seem to offer what caregivers want (p. 48), and so intuitively, it would seem to be a 'good thing'. However, neither this service nor the Geriant model are focused on enablement or stability as such – the emphasis is more on supporting family carers and managing health care problems.

Environmental enablers

Environmental enablers are about 'where' people live and the indoor and outside places in which lives are lived out. These enablers relate to the physical and social environment and can range from minor practical adjustments within the home, such as labelling food cupboards to installing new signage in a neighbourhood to help with wayfinding. For example, an organisation in the Netherlands called Odensehuis provides a meeting room in the local community for people with a dementia to visit. From here there is a grocery route consisting of markings on the pavement from the Odensehuis to the nearby shopping area. This exemplifies environmental enablement as it supports function and creates a sense of stability through material improvements to physical spaces.

Different environments place different demands on a person with a dementia. As disability scholars point out, 'environmental demands require different sets of support elements' (Litvak & Enders, 2001: 725). For example, we know that being in a new and unfamiliar environment (such as a hotel or hospital) can destabilise a person with a dementia. Therefore, support is needed to help the person adjust to the new space. However, familiar environments can be disabling too if the person has no control over or say in how the space is organised. For example, housing association tenants are not always allowed to make modifications to their home even though it may help a person with a dementia who is living there (Lipman & Manthorpe, 2010). An enabling environment is therefore not only about unfamiliarity or familiarity but also being in control.

Research suggests that enabling outdoor environments for people with a dementia are those which people have a long-standing relationship with or at least have a meaningful connection to. This may be because the person is more likely to feel in control in a familiar environment than an unfamiliar one. For example, in a study conducted by Clarke & Bailey (2016) involving 13 families living at home with a dementia, 'belonging and estrangement from place' was found to be a key theme in the data (p. 439). Several participants in the study spoke about the value of living in the same area as there was a 'long-standing familiarity with that place' (p. 443). The study found that familiarity with place can be enabling, and these factors support a 'narrative citizenship' – that is, a continued sense of belonging. Similarly, in the Safer Walking GPS Project, we found that participants who had lived in the same area for many years had a much deeper connection to the community and were able to navigate their way around more easily than those people who had moved recently. Feeling in control is integral then to an enabling environment, and familiar environments are more likely to facilitate that.

Another feature of an enabling environment is that it is a democratic space. Everyone is equal; there are no power imbalances or hierarchies. A coffee shop, restaurant or swimming pool might be thought of in these terms; although it can be anywhere that a person feels they can be themselves, or meet others and have a nice time. In countries nearer the equator, where it is warmer and outside living is the cultural norm, such spaces are likely to be the beach, or in a park or piazza. Sociologists have coined the phrase 'third places' to describe places like this, and they are considered vital for our well-being as they 'provide opportunities for important experiences and relationships in a same society' (Oldenburg, Dennis & Brisset, 1982: 269). For people with a dementia living at home, they can become 'spaces of care' or places of meaning and hope (Bowlby, 2012: 2112).

At this point, we want to clarify what 'place' means, as we have been using it interchangeably with space. Place can be defined as the 'nexus of things within a given boundary' – it has physicality and can be your favourite room, building, village or mountain (O'Toole & Were, 2008: 618). Place is a key characteristic of space; it is the material dimension that simultaneously frames and constitutes social relations (Renedo & Marston, 2015). Thus, we can feel 'at home' in some places but 'out of place' in others. Take, for example, Sion Jair a man aged 67 who has a dementia and lives with his wife in the English Lake District. At the time of writing, Mr Jair was walking and climbing his local mountains twice a day, every single day because he says, 'I found a place where I fit in … I've become part of the landscape and it's become part of me' (Rushby, 2017). Clearly, access to nature and the outdoor environment was enabling Mr Jair to feel good about life.

Other places, such as large towns and cities are likely to have a different impact on a person's lifestyle and spatial preferences. In this situation, a person's citizenship or ethnicity may be central to the story. For instance, in a lovely chapter on people's transitions into communal care, Pooremamali (2017) recounts the story of Hamed (pseudonym) – an 81-year-old man with a dementia from Iraq who had lived in Sweden for more than 20 years. Hamed had always lived in a segregated urban neighbourhood, predominantly with Muslim neighbours, from where he used to enjoy going to the mosque daily in the morning to participate in prayers with his friends (p. 152). For Hamed, the mosque felt like home, which is why he 'felt out of place' in the Swedish care home that he was eventually admitted to. Because the place had no meaning to him, he could not feel a sense of belonging or stability.

A common feature of both these stories is mobility – that is, getting from A to B and experiencing a sense of movement. To have the opportunities to do this is we would suggest is an important environmental enabler. As mobility scholars note, 'movement itself is transformative, changing more than just our relationship with others; it changes our own identities and self of mobilities and personhood too' (Holdsworth, 2013: 23). We have seen how this was the case for both Mr Jair and Hamed. In particular, Mr Jair obviously gains a lot – mentally and physically – from being able to hike long distances in nature. However, the restrictions placed on the movements of people with a dementia often contrasts sharply with how much freedom a person would have had pre-diagnosis – as was the case with Hamed.

Confinement to a particular place or area, whether it is self-imposed or imposed by others, becomes a reality for many people with a dementia, including those who live at home. For example, researchers who used GPS data to compare the 'out-of-home mobility' of people with a mild dementia and healthy controls, found that people with a mild dementia mostly went out in the morning hours and in general had less out-of-home activity than the healthy participants (Shoval et al., 2011: 860). Of even graver concern, another study reports on a woman with a dementia who lived in squalor at the back of her ex-husband's flat: he would let her in and out (Evans et al.,2016). Unless due consideration is given to the mobilities of individuals with a dementia, no environment will be enabling.

The subject of mobility, and in particular transport, comes to the fore when thinking about environmental enablers. From a disability perspective, accessibility is key here – can a person get to where they want to go? Does the person have equal access to services? These are important indicators of an enabling support system, and yet, very few studies have examined the transportation experiences of people with a dementia. Most work has focused on driving cessation rather than access to and use of transport (like mobility scooters, bikes or public transportation systems). When transportation is discussed, it is usually in the context of a wider debate about people's contact with the outside world (see, for example, Genoe, 2009; Brittain, Corner, Robinson, & Bond, 2010). There could more focused attention on people's experiences of transport transitions (e.g. from driver to passenger, travelling in a car to using buses and from pedestrian to mobility scooter user). With this information, we could gain a much fuller picture of the enabling features of a transport system.

In the Safer Walking GPS Project, during the residency people with a dementia and their care partners discussed the difficulties of using public transport. Local buses usually worked quite well, and where these were in quieter areas, such as villages, drivers often got to know the person with a dementia and their family and were able to remind them of their stop when getting off. More complex systems, however, proved exclusionary. There was general agreement that it was impossible for a person with a dementia to get a train ticket from an automated machine. Not only that so much information was required quickly, but the pressure from other passengers wanting to get tickets quickly precluded taking adequate time to work it out. Having a person to buy a ticket from was much more enticing, but many small stations do not have that facility. Providing communities that are dementia enabled will require rethinking about how public transport systems are designed to support people with a dementia to use them.

Structural enablers

Structural enablers are about 'how' to create the optimum socio-political environment for people with a dementia to live at home. Structural enablers aim to support function and create a sense of stability through legislation, national initiatives and plans, as well new funding schemes. Countries such as India and those in the Asia–Pacific region offer clear examples of structural enablers as they use socio-legal frameworks to encourage people to live in a particular way. For example, the 'Senior Citizens Act 2007' in India gives tax relief to families who care for elderly relatives but applies penalties to those families who avoid their responsibilities (Brijnath, 2012: 698). In Singapore, government statutes are used to socially engineer children either to live together or to live within a short distance of their elderly parents and/or parents-in-law. More recently in China, a new law came into effect in 2013 – the Protection of the Rights and Interests of the Elderly People – which requires adult children to visit and care for their ageing parents on a regular basis. Such legislation may seem tough;

however, given the size of the population in China – in 2006, 8% of the country's 1.3 billion people were aged 65 or above, and this percentage is expected to increase to 24% by 2050 (Chiu, Yu, & Lam, 2010) – it is likely to be extremely difficult to enforce.

Another 'gentler' example of a structural enabler is the 'Dementia Friendly Communities' (DFC) movement. This seeks to improve the general environment for people with a dementia on a global scale by raising awareness and enhancing societal understanding of people's needs and rights. The World Health Organization urges countries throughout the world to have at least one DFC by 2025 to foster a 'dementia-inclusive' society. Communities are recognised as 'dementia friendly' when they meet certain criteria, including plans for raising awareness. The UK is a forerunner with developing DFCs – there are over 200 recognised DFCs in England and Wales alone. However, it is a global movement and countries across the world are developing DFCs (Alzheimer's Disease International, 2015). While such widespread action is encouraging, the notion of 'dementia friendly' has been criticised for its patronising tone and risk of creating a 'them and us' divide; hence, there are calls for an assets-based approach (Rahman & Swaffer, 2018). Arguably, though, an equally pressing priority is to establish whether DFCs are enabling people with a dementia to live at home.

As well as developing DFCs, many countries have in place or are drafting a national plan for dementia. These plans have similar themes, such as improving community support and improving assessment and diagnostic practices and often involve the active engagement of people with a dementia in their development. For example, at the time of writing this the Welsh Government had just completed its consultation on its draft strategy entitled: 'Together for a Dementia Friendly Wales 2017–22' and the Netherlands had launched its five-year campaign 'Together we make the Netherlands Dementia Friendly'. Clearly, more and more countries are working in a strategic way to create the right environment for people with a dementia and their families to gain the support they need to live well with a dementia.

Governments are keen to create the optimum socio-political environment for people with a dementia to live at home, not only but because that is what most people want, but because of the rising costs of providing care. As one analyst points out, 'the choice between "home care" or specialized establishments is deeply structured in terms of values but also in financial terms' (Long Term coverage in Europe (2015: 18). As a result, different countries will have different approaches to funding. For example, in Iceland – where citizens are entitled by law to round-the-clock social and health services – the government has started to regulate access to care homes due to the escalating costs of institutional care (Björnsdóttir, Ceci, & Purkis, 2015). As these authors explain, Iceland had the highest proportion of institutional placements for older people in the Nordic countries and the median time that a person lived in a nursing home (3.5 years) was higher compared to the other countries (p. 67). The regulation sought to ensure all available community-based options had been utilised before care in a long-term care facility was funded. In contrast, in the UK, NHS commissioning groups are unlikely to fund home care for an older person who requires more than eight hours of care at home, as institutional care is regarded as a more cost-effective long-term option. Fundamentally then, enabling life at home raises a big economic question for governments, households and individuals alike – who pays for it? We return to this question in the concluding chapter.

Conclusion

The account of enabling life at home we have offered in this chapter attempts to challenge some existing viewpoints on the topic of community-based support and services. By focusing on the perspective of the person with a dementia and making life at home liveable we have highlighted some of the ways in which enablement might be possible. We have deliberately used an idea from disability studies of 'enabling support systems' in an effort to enter the medical trope of 'caregiver burden' for a more civilised and caring way of thinking about life at home for people with a dementia and their supporters.

References

Alwin, J., Öberg, B., & Krevers, B. (2010). Support/services among family caregivers of persons with dementia: Perceived importance and services received. *International Journal of Geriatric Psychiatry, 25*(3), 240–248. https://doi.org/10.1002/gps.2328

Antelius, E. (2017). Dementia in the age of migration: Cross cultural perspectives. In L.-C. Hydén & E. Antelius (Eds.), *Living with Dementia: Relations, Responses and Agency in Everyday Life*. London: Palgrave Macmillan.

Banerjee, S. (2015). Multimorbidity: Older adults need health care that can count past one. *The Lancet, 385*(9968), 587–589. https://doi.org/10.1016/S0140-6736(14)61596-8

Banerjee, S., Murray, J., Foley, B., Atkins, L., Schneider, J., & Mann, A. (2003). Predictors of institutionalisation in people with dementia. *Journal of Neurology, Neurosurgery, and Psychiatry, 74*(9), 1315–1316. https://doi.org/10.1136/JNNP.74.9.1315

Björnsdóttir, K., Ceci, C., & Purkis, M. E. (2015). The 'right' place to care for older people: Home or institution? *Nursing Inquiry, 22*(1), 64–73. https://doi.org/10.1111/nin.12041

Bowlby, S. (2012). Recognising the time-space dimensions of care: Caringscapes and carescapes. *Environment and Planning A, 44*(9), 2101–2118. https://doi.org/10.1068/a44492

Boyle, G. (2014). 'Can't cook, won't cook': Men's involvement in cooking when their wives develop dementia. *Journal of Gender Studies, 23*(4), 336–350. https://doi.org/10.1080/09589236.2013.792728

Brijnath, B. (2012). Why does institutionalised care not appeal to Indian families? Legislative and social answers from urban India. *Ageing and Society, 32*(4), 697–717. https://doi.org/10.1017/S0144686X11000584

Brittain, K., Corner, L., Robinson, L., & Bond, J. (2010). Ageing in place and technologies of place: The lived experience of people with dementia in changing social, physical and technological environments. *Sociology of Health & Illness, 32*(2), 272–87. https://doi.org/10.1111/j.1467-9566.2009.01203.x

Bunn, F., Goodman, C., Pinkney, E., & Drennan, V. M. (2016). Specialist nursing and community support for the carers of people with dementia living at home: An evidence synthesis. *Health and Social Care in the Community, 24*(1), 48–67. https://doi.org/10.1111/hsc.12189

Chiu, H. F. K., Yu, X., & Lam, L. C. W. (2010). Dementia strategy in China and Hong Kong. *International Journal of Geriatric Psychiatry, 25*(9), 905–907. https://doi.org/10.1002/gps.2595

CIHI. (2017). *Seniors in Transition: Exploring Pathways Across the Care Continuum*. https://www.cihi.ca/en/seniors-in-transition-exploring-pathways-across-the-care-continuum

Clarke, C. L., & Bailey, C. (2016). Narrative citizenship, resilience and inclusion with dementia: On the inside or on the outside of physical and social places. *Dementia, 15*(3), 434–452. https://doi.org/10.1177/1471301216639736

Eriksen, S., Helvik, A. S., Juvet, L. K., Skovdahl, K., Førsund, L. H., & Grov, E. K. (2016). The experience of relations in persons with dementia: A systematic meta-synthesis. *Dementia and Geriatric Cognitive Disorders, 42*(5–6), 342–368. https://doi.org/10.1159/000452404

Evans, D., Price, K., & Meyer, J. (2016). Home alone with dementia. *SAGE Open, 6*(3), 1–13. https://doi.org/10.1177/2158244016664954

Genoe, M. R. (2009). *Living with hope in the midst of change: The meaning of leisure within the context of dementia*. PhD Thesis. University of Waterloo.

Glimmerveen, L., & Nies, H. (2015). Community-based dementia care: The Geriant model. *International Journal of Integrated Care, 15*(September), 1–15. https://doi.org/http://doi.org/10.5334/ijic.1796

Hales, G. (1996). *Beyond Disability: Towards an Enabling Society*. London: Sage Publications.

Hayes, J., Boylstein, C., & Zimmerman, M. K. (2009). Living and loving with dementia: Negotiating spousal and caregiver identity through narrative. *Journal of Aging Studies, 23*(1), 48–59. https://doi.org/10.1016/j.jaging.2007.09.002

Hellström, I., & Larsson, A. T. (2017). Dementia as chronic illness: Maintaining involvement in everyday life. In L.-C. Hydén & E. Antelius (Eds.), *Living with Dementia: Relations, Responses and Agency in Everyday Life* (pp. 136–148). London: Palgrave Macmillan.

Holdsworth, C. (2013). *Family and Intimate Mobilities*. Basingstoke: Palgrave Macmillan.

Kane, M., & Cook, L. (2013). Dementia 2013: The hidden voice of loneliness (April). London: *Alzheimer's Society*, iii–64.

Lipman, V., & Manthorpe, J. (2010). Gearing up. London: Age UK. www.utilities-me.com

Lister, R. (2007). Inclusive citizenship: Realizing the potential. *Citizenship Studies, 11*(1), 49–61. https://doi.org/10.1080/13621020601099856

Litvak, S., & Enders, A. (2001). Support systems: The interface between individuals and environments. In Albrecht, G. L., Seelman, K. D., & Bury, M. (Eds.), *Handbook of Disability Studies* (pp. 711–732). California: Sage Publications.

Lord, K., Livingston, G., Robertson, S., & Cooper, C. (2016). How people with dementia and their families decide about moving to a care home and support their needs: Development of a decision aid, a qualitative study. *BMC Geriatrics, 16*(1), 68. https://doi.org/10.1186/s12877-016-0242-1

Mendes, A. (2015). Intergenerational work: Putting the magic back into dementia care. *Nursing and Residential Care, 17*(12), 692–694.

Moriarty, B. J., Sharif, N., & Robinson, J. (2011). Black and minority ethnic people with dementia and their access to support and services (March). London: Social Care Institute for Excellence.

National Housing Federation & HACT (2015). Transforming care pathways for people with dementia: Linking housing, health and social care (October). London: National Housing Federation & HACT.

Oldenburg, D., & Brisset, R. (1982). The third place. *Qualitative Sociology, 5*(4), 265–284. https://doi.org/10.1007/BF00986754

O'Rourke, H. M., Duggleby, W., Fraser, K. D., & Jerke, L. (2015). Factors that affect quality of life from the perspective of people with dementia: A metasynthesis. *Journal of the American Geriatrics Society, 63*(1), 24–38. https://doi.org/10.1111/jgs.13178

Orpin, P., Stirling, C., Hetherington, S., & Robinson, A. (2012). Rural dementia carers: Formal and informal sources of support. *Ageing and Society, 34*(2), 1–24. https://doi.org/10.1017/S0144686X12000827

O'Toole, P., & Were, P. (2008). Observing places: Using space and material culture in qualitative research. *Qualitative Research, 8*(5), 616–634. https://doi.org/10.1177/1468794108093899

Phillipson, L., Magee, C., & Jones, S. C. (2013). Why carers of people with dementia do not utilise out-of-home respite services. *Health and Social Care in the Community, 21*(4), 411–422. https://doi.org/10.1111/hsc.12030

Pols, J. (2017). How to make your relationship work? Aesthetic relations with technology. *Foundations of Science, 22*(2), 421–424. https://doi.org/10.1007/s10699-015-9449-4

Pooremamali, P. (2017). 'Home is somewhere in-between-passage': The stories of relocation to a residential home by persons with dementia. In E. Hyden & L.-C. Antelius (Eds.), *Living with Dementia: Relations, Responses and Agency in Everyday Life* (pp. 149–164). London: Palgrave Macmillan.

Rahman, S., & Swaffer, K. (2018). Assets-based approaches and dementia-friendly communities. *Dementia, 17*(2), 131–137. http://journals.sagepub.com/doi/10.1177/1471301217751533

Renedo, A., & Marston, C. (2015). Spaces for citizen involvement in healthcare: An ethnographic study. *Sociology, 49*(3), 488–504. https://doi.org/10.1177/0038038514544208

Rushby, K. (2017, May 5). Mountains of the mind: 'I've become part of the landscape and it's become part of me'. *The Guardian.*

Shaw, S., Rosen, R., & Rumbold, B. (2011). What is integrated care? Research report (June). London: *Nuffield Trust*, 1–23.

Shoval, N., Wahl, H.-W., Auslander, G., Isaacson, M., Oswald, F., Edry, T., Heinik, J. (2011). Use of the global positioning system to measure the out-of-home mobility of older adults with differing cognitive functioning. *Ageing and Society, 31*(5), 849–869. https://doi.org/10.1017/S0144686X10001455

Singleton, D., Mukadam, N., Livingston, G., & Sommerlad, A. (2017). How people with dementia and carers understand and react to social functioning changes in mild dementia: A UK-based qualitative study. *BMJ Open, 7*(7), e016740. https://doi.org/10.1136/bmjopen-2017-016740

Smebye, K. L., Kirkevold, M., & Engedal, K. (2012). How do persons with dementia participate in decision making related to health and daily care? A multi-case study. *BMC Health Services Research, 12*(1), 241. https://doi.org/10.1186/1472-6963-12-241

Smebye, K. L., Kirkevold, M., & Engedal, K. (2016). Ethical dilemmas concerning autonomy when persons with dementia wish to live at home: A qualitative, hermeneutic study. *BMC Health Services Research, 16*(1), 21. https://doi.org/10.1186/s12913-015-1217-1

Vandepitte, S., Van Den Noortgate, N., Putman, K., Verhaeghe, S., & Annemans, L. (2016). Effectiveness and cost-effectiveness of an in-home respite care program in supporting informal caregivers of people with dementia: Design of a comparative study. *BMC Geriatrics, 16*(1), 207. https://doi.org/10.1186/s12877-016-0373-4

Verbeek, H., Meyer, G., Leino-Kilpi, H., Zabalegui, A., Hallberg, I. R., Saks, K., … Hamers, J. P. H. (2012). A European study investigating patterns of transition from home care towards institutional dementia care: The protocol of a RightTimePlaceCare study. *BMC Public Health, 12*(1), 68. https://doi.org/10.1186/1471-2458-12-68

Verbrugge, L. M., & Jette, A. M. (1994). The disablement process. *Social Science and Medicine, 38*(1), 1–14. https://doi.org/10.1016/0277-9536(94)90294-1

von Kutzleben, M., Reuther, S., Dortmann, O., & Holle, B. (2016). Care arrangements for community-dwelling people with dementia in Germany as perceived by informal carers – a cross-sectional pilot survey in a provincial-rural setting. *Health and Social Care in the Community, 24*(3), 283–296. https://doi.org/10.1111/hsc.12202

Winter, L., Gitlin, L. N., & Dennis, M. (2011). Desire to institutionalize a relative with dementia: Quality of premorbid relationship and caregiver gender. *Family Relations, 60*(2), 221–230. https://doi.org/10.1111/j.1741-3729.2010.00644.x

Worth, N. (2013). Making friends and fitting in: A social-relational understanding of disability at school. *Social & Cultural Geography, 14*(1), 103–123. https://doi.org/10.1080/14649365.2012.735693

Wu, C., Gao, L., & Dong, H. (2016). Care services for elderly people with dementia in rural China: A case study (November 2015). *World Health Organization,* 167–173. https://doi.org/10.2471/BLT.15.160929

4

RETHINKING SELF-MANAGEMENT

Introduction

Self-management is about someone with a health condition maintaining themselves and staying well for as long as they possibly can. It requires a person to understand and manage their own condition and treatment and to know when and who to ask for help. Conventionally, self-management includes some level of self-monitoring and treatment with medication, as is the case with someone diagnosed with diabetes. However, it is increasingly used to describe a broad spectrum of activities that a person might engage in to stay well, such as taking physical exercise to manage a mental health problem. The idea of self-management is applied to people with a dementia living at home, and it is suggested that it requires a relational component to be meaningful for this group. This is because, while self-care may be an achievable and desirable aim for some people with a dementia, it will not be possible for everyone, all of the time. As the condition progresses and the effects of dementia become more severe, the ability to self-manage will become more and more precarious and eventually impossible. This chapter critiques the concept of self-management in relation to people with a dementia and develops an understanding that is more relational in quality – relational care of selves. This considers that independence and self-care are important to people with a dementia, but this is best placed alongside the care from and of others. In developing this new way of thinking about self-management, we examine who needs to be involved, rather than what needs to be done in order for people with a dementia to live well. Piette and Arbor (2010) recognise the essential role of family caregivers and other kin in promoting the well-being of people with long-term conditions, and we adopt that thinking to consider how self-management needs to be adapted. Furthermore, we draw on ideas from Eastern cultures, where collectivism and mutualism have more currency than autonomy.

In this chapter, self-management, as it applies to dementia, is critiqued, and we consider why an alternative concept would be beneficial to the lives of people with a dementia. Notwithstanding that people with a dementia may welcome some aspects of self-management, such as being proactive about health management to stay as independent as possible for as long as possible. This is likely to face increasing challenges as dementia and potentially other long-term conditions progress. Self-management refers to the responsibility of health management by an individual, maintaining or improving health through control over a variety of daily activities, including diet, exercise and treatment adherence. We suggest that a relational approach is more fitting – a relational care of selves, which is extended to consider self-care and care for each other for people with a dementia and those involved in their care. The boxed text in this chapter is from John and Fiona, who responded to our ideas about self-management.

We examine self-management and dementia, using a critical approach to consider how appropriate self-management is given the current state of knowledge about dementia and how it impacts on people. Then we consider self-management in its more familiar territory – in type 2 diabetes mellitus and how a person with a dementia may negotiate this condition. Finally, we consider relational care of selves by considering a shared activity where care for each other and the self are recognised for people with a dementia and those who care for them.

Dementia and self-management

Dementia is an umbrella term that refers to numerous syndromes such as Alzheimer's disease, Lewy Body dementia, Pick's disease, Vascular dementia, Frontotemporal Lobe dementia, Primary Progressive Aphasia, Creutzfelt–Jacob disease and Huntington's Chorea. Mixed dementia is a form of dementia that has characteristics from at least two types of these dementias. Common symptoms of dementia, such as memory loss and disorganisation, may feature in other long-term conditions such as Parkinson's disease. Each type of dementia has an expected disease trajectory; however, the experience of dementia may be very different between individuals with similar types. Evidence of how dementias affect individuals continues to emerge, as discussed in earlier chapters of this book.

Dementia does not fit neatly into the medical model because of the gaps in knowledge about causes, treatment and prognosis. Generally, for each of the dementias (except Huntington's Chorea, which has a known genetic cause and no cure) the medical understanding looks like this:

- Aetiology   Some hypotheses
- Cause   Some hypotheses are being tested
- Diagnosis   Unclear, testing has improved
- Treatment   No curative treatment; medication slows progress
- Prognosis   Unpredictable

Self-management works best when measurable symptoms influence treatment options, such as a blood glucose reading, influencing calorific intake or insulin dose. It is essential to note that because of the lack of measurable symptoms of dementia, the promotion of self-management is nebulous. Self-management in dementia is not a calibration of the illness; there are no measurements that can be taken that inform medical treatment or other interventions. Rather, it is an attempt to decrease the impact of the disease on daily functioning. Limited studies on the usefulness of self-management to people in the early stages of dementia found that it was the togetherness of the group that helped people manage better (Quinn et al., 2014; 2016; Toms, Quinn, Anderson, & Clare, 2015). In many aspects of health care, emphasis is now placed on the individual as responsible for health management and, where possible, improvement.

Self-management is concerned with how the individual negotiates a long-term condition, acts on knowledge of the condition, avoids behaviours that may worsen the condition and adheres to the advice of clinical practitioners. For example, according to Kirk et al. (2015) self-management of type 2 diabetes mellitus includes, once daily self-foot checks; consuming fruits and vegetables (at least five servings per day five or more times per week); participation in exercise (five or more times per week); once daily self-monitoring of blood glucose; professional foot check at least twice during the year, or HbA1c blood check at least twice over the year; alongside daily self-care activities that include diet and exercise. Thus, there is a lot of work involved.

Self-management commonly consists of education about the condition, control of behaviours that affect the condition and compliance with medical and clinical advice to promote better health (Mountain, 2017). To achieve this, collaboration between the service user and clinician is required, recognising the service user as an expert on their condition (Bodenheimer, Lorig, Holman, & Grumbach, 2002). Lorig and Holman (2003: 1) suggest that a person who has a long-term condition 'cannot not manage' it. Everyday decisions about diet, activity and exercise are reconstructed as health and wellness decisions that influence the course and prognosis of the long-term condition. Eating, exercise and taking medication all form self-management behaviours that health professionals give advice about but that the public may ignore:

> Patients are in control. No matter what we as health professionals do or say, patients are in control of these important self-management decisions. When patients leave the clinic or office, they can and do veto recommendations a health professional makes.
>
> *(Bodenheimer et al., 2002: 2469)*

People influence their control over the condition either by engaging with knowledge and advice and make judgements about what will improve their situation or by neglecting to focus on it. A significant criticism is that the expectation of self-management foregrounds the illness above all else in the person's life to an extent that may not be achievable in the daily bustle of meeting one's needs.

The issue of self-management is further complicated when it is considered that many people with a dementia have one or more coexisting long-term conditions to manage as well. These may include mobility and/or sensory impairments, long-term pain, mental health issues and common physical health conditions that affect older people such as diabetes or heart problems. Complications arise when it may be difficult to locate the interplay of each of these conditions or the impacts of polypharmacy. This complication can be intensified by the lack of awareness that practitioners who have knowledge of other long-term conditions have about dementias. Notwithstanding these complications, people with a dementia may be encouraged to self-manage, and in the next section the ideas underpinning self-management will be critiqued and a more fitting set of principles for people with a dementia will be discussed. Later in the chapter, we examine the specific challenges of living with a dementia and diabetes and attempting to self-manage both. We conclude by suggesting that self-management as a concept would be strengthened in relation to dementia if it were conceptually developed alongside people with a dementia as part of the further research needed on the topic.

Self-management emerged from grassroots responses to health and social issues, such as self-help groups established to offer peer support. These groups were coterminous to health and social care established by experts by experience, who shared that expertise with others (Ward, 2015). This was necessary as health services do not provide this kind of detailed experiential knowledge (Scott, 2011). Despite these origins, self-management more usually refers to individual-ised responsibility and compliance with clinical assessment and treatment, and, as raised earlier, this is most effective where the medical response is clear and effec-tive. Boger et al. (2015) conducted a systematic review of stakeholders' desired outcomes from the practice of self-management and found that the evidence was unclear as there was little attention paid to stakeholders' views about what con-stituted important outcomes. This makes the specific aims of self-management unclear, but behaviours associated with self-management are open to judgement. Ellis et al. (2017: 28) identified three traits of the *good self-manager* from their study of physical long-term health conditions, which can be seen in Figure 4.1.

Here, these are discussed in relation to the self-management of dementia.

Trait one: Remoralised – being responsible; fulfilling moral obligations

Taking responsibility includes everyday actions that promote health such as eating well and exercising, not smoking and not drinking excessive alcohol. In dementia, this may be extended to memory training or other strategies to manage impacts. Asking most people if, in the last week, they have managed to eat seven to ten portions of fruit and vegetables a day, exercise for one hour a day (recommended in New Zealand), not smoke and drink alcohol within recommended limits, it may be a limited number of people who do so. This idealised lifestyle has been significantly criticised as over-simplified, such as through the influence of

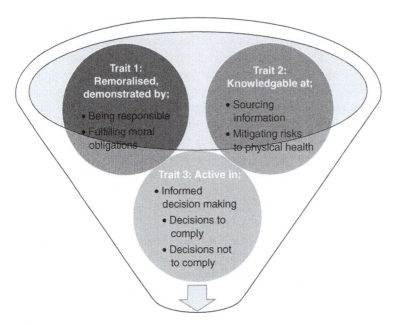

FIGURE 4.1 The 'good' self-manager

obesogenic environments where fast food is abundant, resulting in higher obesity rates in some neighbourhoods more than others (Harrington & Elliot, 2009). Numerous factors interfere with the ability to live a healthy life. These include psychological motivation or that time and resources may be limited due to caring responsibilities.

Taking responsibility for a dementia is often interpreted as an individual level of responsibility for forestalling the development of a dementia. Ascribing this kind of responsibility alongside the challenge of dementia does not help people to live well. Promoting healthier lifestyles may well decrease the impacts of long-term conditions across the lifespan but it will not guarantee against dementia. Likewise, cognitive training and brain games do not forestall or prevent dementia (Ratner & Atkinson, 2015) despite the widespread acceptance that they do.

BOX 4.1 JOHN: *I WOULD LIKE A NEW BRAIN*

We discussed the slogan that is often attached to dementia, 'Use it or Lose it'. John thought that it would be like that – use it or lose it – but it absolutely was not. He tries really hard to learn and remember new things, but they escape him, and he cannot remember them. John has great determination to do new things, but even with that determination and wanting to do it, he is unable to. Some people try to be very encouraging with the mantra 'come on, you can do it'. But John says he simply cannot do it and that 'if I ask for help, I need it'. Fiona and John had a recent visitor who suggested that they concentrate on what John can do, not what he can't. When John was asked what he thought about this, he was not sure. He thought about it and said, *I can go out for a walk. Apart from that, there aren't really very many things that I can do without help.*

There is currently little emphasis on the need for people with a dementia to continue with health-promoting behaviours after diagnosis, or physical health checks to promote health. An example from the Safer Walking GPS Project is that of a man in his 50s diagnosed with a dementia. He is a keen cyclist and in discussion with his friends and local gym, a cycling group was set up so that he may be chaperoned while out cycling so as not to get lost. A local large international company heard about this and agreed to support his cycling by volunteering a cyclist to accompany him once a week. Another example, however, was a woman in her forties who was a keen runner but because she was afraid of getting lost, and no intervention was available, she had stopped running.

BOX 4.2 BEING WITH FAMILY MAKES MY 'HEART SING'

We discussed what John thinks supports his well-being, what challenges his well-being and what makes his heart sing. Without hesitation, John mentioned that Fiona and having his family around makes his heart sing. He enjoys walking and staying mobile is a priority. He continues to enjoy going to the rugby with friends. John experiences anxiety and this really challenges his well-being. The anxiety has worsened, and he has discussed it with his doctor to see if he can get some treatment. John described fearing how the dementia is progressing and notices things he is no longer able to do, things that he used to be able to do without a thought.

Trait two: Knowledgeable – sourcing information; mitigating risks to (physical) health.

Sourcing information

Information about how to manage is most often available through advocacy organisations such as the Alzheimer's Society. The major symptoms of a dementia are well rehearsed, such as memory loss or loss of organisational skills, but how the illness will impact on each person is largely unpredictable. More accounts of living with a dementia are becoming available, and these provide insights for others about key issues, such as sharing the diagnosis, disclosing dementia to families, transitions of identity and relationships. But also, each family finds its own way.

Families who support a person with a dementia by encouraging (not criticising) and supporting (not undermining) have a greater chance of enabling the person with a dementia to have a good sense of well-being (see for example the University of Bradford 2008 well-being profile based on Kitwood's [1990] principles). People with a dementia and their families who accept that cognitive acuity is not the zenith of existence and that there are other skills and talents that continue to be useful and relevant, tend to fare better in their well-being than others. The stereotype of the intellectual person, such as authors and academics, feeds into the public imaginary as those most tragically struck by dementia (see, for example, the film *Still Alice* 2014).

As each person with a dementia and their family find their way, solutions to difficulties are found through peer support, such as dementia cafes, singing groups and internet groups. The Alzheimer's Society has a lively forum, Talking Point, where people share problems and ideas. This sharing of ground-up knowledge is essential to finding the answers to the challenges of dementia, reflecting the origin of the self-help group.

In the Safer Walking GPS Project, people with a dementia and carers discussed the challenges of accessing the right information at the right time. For some, the diagnosis was welcomed and medications accepted, with visits to the memory clinic every six months. Being active and healthy was a common goal. However, the future was always unknown and questions hung in the air, such as to how do I know what is coming and when and how can I plan for the unknown. Many people asked us how they seemed, and whether they were doing okay.

Mitigating risks

Risk is predominantly conceptualised as the increased level of risk presented by the person with a dementia who is unaware of their actions being risky. High levels of risk that signify increased vulnerability, such as inviting strangers into the home or going out alone at night, are associated with residential placement (Ledgerd et al., 2015). Less often is it considered that people with a dementia mitigate risks as they occur to them, or that people with a dementia may take positive risks to maintain being active. One of the participants in the Safer Walking GPS Project described how, having struggled to remember how to get home when out alone, had decided the best approach was 'safety first'. He limited going out to when others would be able to go with him, or only going out on very well-known routes to avoid getting into any difficulty. Limiting his risk involved staying indoors and occupying himself watching television, whilst others did not understand why he was not going out to maintain his social activity and physical health. He explained that it was not possible to continue to be brought home by others. When he had got into difficulties he had sat calmly in the village where he lived and asked someone (who he would often know) for help, and had always got home safely.

Many people with a dementia talk about the anxiety of not feeling in control – an uncertainty that is often unknown to them previously. Going out, people may fear appearing vulnerable, for example, using money or bank cards. People with a dementia may not formally be assessed for risk, such as road safety, safety around the house, or going out without informing others. Some people with a dementia may also not recognise that they are at risk and may not accept or perceive risks that others see. For some, this may be linked to cognitive decline and an inability to satisfactorily assess and judge a situation. Mitigating risk is likely to take into consideration these feelings of loss of control, and therefore to limit what is tried or to do things differently. This new dependence can have quite a demand on close family members, going from doing things alone to relying on others.

Trait three: Active in informed decision-making; decisions to comply; decisions not to comply

For people with a dementia to be active in informed decision-making the availability, timing and accessibility of relevant information and the facilitation of inclusion are needed. Information presented in an accessible format, at a relevant time, will enable people to contribute if they can. Making sense of information in context is helpful. Abstracted decisions are harder to grasp, so creating scenarios that detail the context with possible decisions helps people with a dementia to contribute.

Once information is provided in an accessible and timely fashion, people with a dementia have a right to make their own decision, whether in agreement with others or not. That people with a dementia may lack the ability to make a decision is not questioned – this may be a reality as dementia advances – however, where people are able to make a decision, it is how the person is facilitated to do so that counts (Fetherstonhaugh, Tarzia, & Nay, 2013). It is suggested that in care situations, all contributors are asked to state preferred outcomes, including clinicians, family members and people who are cared for. An example in relation to self-management is where a person with a dementia lives at home with their partner who needs a break. The person with a dementia is reluctant to attend a day centre. The following is a list of all the preferences that need to be taken into account:

- Family member – wants the person with a dementia to attend a day centre at least twice a week to be able to get a rest as they are not sleeping very well because the person with a dementia gets up at night and disturbs their sleep.
- Person with a dementia – does not want to go to a day centre that is full of other people with a dementia as they find it really depressing. Has visited and there is little to do there that is stimulating and many of the other attendees are much older and have more advanced dementia.

- Dementia adviser – can see that the partner needs a rest, and if the partner is not able to continue caring, the person with a dementia is likely to have to be placed in residential care. Has discussed other strategies for getting better sleep but partner has not taken any of them up.
- Other family members – want person with a dementia to 'behave' and support partner by doing what they are told.
- GP – has suggested night sedation for person with a dementia, which has not been tried.

Here, it would be helpful to have an agreed aim, such as to help the person with a dementia remain at home and several possible interventions. One supportive approach would be to examine all possibilities for the person with a dementia to be occupied in a way that is more acceptable to them. This may include alternatives to the day centre or supported introductions to other activities. A thorough and careful assessment would explore and examine a variety of ways of better meeting both sets of needs.

In summary, there are significant challenges to the achievement of self-management by people with a dementia. Health is influenced across the life course, with those getting a better start in life being in a better position to achieve good health and healthy behaviours across the lifespan are continued in later life. Once people get a diagnosis of a dementia, often health-promoting activities are not factored as important and people do not get the help they need to access them. Where people are motivated to look after themselves, to eat well and exercise and stay as well as possible, they should be encouraged and facilitated to do so. We suggest that a systematic approach to logging the preferences and potential outcomes becomes part of practice to enable those preferences of people with a dementia to be recognised and the outcomes stated in terms of whose needs they meet.

Self-managing dementia and type 2 diabetes mellitus

Another common long-term health condition is diabetes of which there are two main types, type 1 diabetes and type 2 diabetes. Type 1 diabetes affects between 5 and 15% of people with diabetes and is usually diagnosed in people under 30 years but can affect people of any age. Type 1 diabetes is treated with insulin injections, a healthy eating plan and regular physical activity. Type 2 diabetes is more common in older people and affects 85–90% of people with diabetes (Hill et al., 2013). Longitudinal studies show a relationship between cognitive impairment and type 2 diabetes and is the predominant type of diabetes in people with a dementia (Allen, Frier, & Strachan, 2004).

Type 2 diabetes is associated with a 1.5 to twofold higher risk of dementia (Sinclair, Hilison, & Bayer, 2014). As we know, dementia is typically characterised by progressive and significant changes to executive functions including memory, language, reasoning and thinking, as well as other adverse effects such as changes in personality and visual–perceptual problems. All these attributes affect the ability to recognise and report the signs and symptoms of diabetes and subsequently self-manage the condition. Like type 2 diabetes, the risk of developing dementia increases rapidly with age; both dementia and type 2 diabetes mellitus are common long-term disabling conditions and may inevitably co-exist in a significant number of older people by the very fact of their high prevalence rates. For instance, a cross-sectional analysis of 497,900 US veterans with diabetes found that 8% of participants aged 65–74 also had a dementia, and 5% had a cognitive impairment (Feil et al., 2011b).

The evidence from large-scale studies on managing diabetes in people with a dementia suggests that effective management and support is key to the prevention of cognitive decline and related problems. For example, one Randomised Controlled Trial conducted in the United States found an association between improved diabetes control in older people and less global cognitive decline (Luchsinger et al., 2011). Another community-based case-control study conducted in Wales found an association between low score on the Mini-Mental State Examination (suggestive of poor cognition) and poorer ability in diabetes self-care, greater dependency and higher hospitalisation (Sinclair, Girling, & Bayer, 2000). However, it is not clear to what extent a lack of self-management and poor health outcomes are linked.

Managing type 2 diabetes effectively is essential for good health and well-being, particularly so for people with cognitive impairment or a dementia as sub-optimal management can exacerbate an already deleterious situation. For example, evidence derived from a trial indicates that improved type 2 diabetes control can delay global decline in people aged 55 years and over (Luchsinger et al., 2011). This study tested the effectiveness of a type 2 diabetes case management intervention, which involved a home telemedicine unit consisting of a web-enabled computer with modern connection to an existing telephone line to allow for video conferencing with nurse care managers at a type 2 diabetes clinic (Shea et al., 2009). The researchers found the intervention improved glycated haemoglobin, systolic blood pressure and LDL-cholesterol, which in turn delayed cognitive decline (Luchsinger et al., 2011: 447). However, this study and other research evaluating the effectiveness of interventions raises questions about how such strategies might work for people with a dementia who live at home.

People with a dementia who live at home are likely to face considerable challenges when it comes to managing type 2 diabetes as they are less likely to have someone to prompt or support them to do the tasks they need to do to stay well. Take, for instance, one of the respondents in a qualitative study conducted by Wilson (2012) who lived alone; she reported being admitted to hospital because she had no one to remind her to check her blood glucose or take insulin. This case highlights the risk of hypoglycaemia in older people and people with a dementia, especially those who live alone. As Sinclair, Hilison and Bayer (2014) point out, 'people with a pre-existing diagnosis of diabetes who are subsequently diagnosed with a dementia may find their "hypo" awareness is comprised as their cognitive function deteriorates'.

Quality of life is often linked to the ability to self-manage in diabetes care. Being empowered to look after oneself (i.e. test blood glucose, exercise, eat a healthy diet, inspect feet, carry diabetes identification, go for regular health checks) is increasingly seen as fundamental to the well-being of people with diabetes (Acce, 2012). For example, one study based on interviews with older people with cognitive impairment or a dementia sheds light on the strategies that individuals and families use to manage diabetes. This research, based on qualitative interviews involving 25 people aged between 72 and 84 years with either type 1 or type 2 diabetes, found that older people with type 2 diabetes have 'varying diabetes management skills and coping strategies that they may have performed for years to accommodate the disease in their lifestyle' (Wilson, 2012: 37). It should not be assumed, therefore, that everyone with a dementia will necessarily be managing type 2 diabetes for the first time, although some people will.

One perspective that tends to be missing in the research literature is the view of individuals personally affected by these conditions. Living with diabetes can be hard work (Nash, 2013), especially if you have a dementia, yet attention is typically paid to the challenges it creates for doctors, clinicians and family caregivers (see, for example, Feil, Lukman, Simon, Walston, & Vickery, 2011a). The neglect of direct evidence from the person with a dementia is a feature of the general research literature on the impact of caring for a person with a dementia (Ablitt, Jones, & Muers, 2009). One particular risk for people with both diabetes and a dementia is that their best interests and rights are overshadowed by those of the carers. For example, research shows that people with type 2 diabetes and cognitive problems may not be involved in decisions concerning their care and may feel excluded, especially if those around them seek to over-manage or over-control the situation due to concerns about risk (Wilson, 2012). Guidance on positive risk-taking, while not specifically about the challenges associated with managing type 2 diabetes in people with a dementia, acknowledges that people with a dementia have other illnesses and may lose their independence if a broad approach to risk management is not taken by all involved (DoH, 2010). As such, the proposed work will contribute to broader policymaking and implementation related to positive risk-taking and people with a dementia (DoH, 2010).

Practical guidance on managing type 2 diabetes in people with a dementia is available, but it is aimed at clinicians rather than those living with the condition. This literature sets out the range of clinical issues associated with type 2 diabetes and a dementia in older people and provides practical guidance on the principles of type 2 diabetes management for those diagnosed with a dementia. These are to:

- review a person's ability to self-manage regularly;
- consider problems of adherence to medication and simplify medication regimens wherever possible;

- prescribe glucose lowering medications with a low risk of causing hypoglycaemia wherever possible;
- review nutritional status;
- ensure appropriate control of all vascular risk factors such as blood pressure and cholesterol levels;
- recognise the terminal phase of severe dementia and modify medications accordingly
- provide appropriate support to informal carers.

(Hill et al., 2013: 12)

From this example, it is possible to see how complex and problematic the notion of self-management is for people with a dementia.

Relational care of selves

Self-management is problematic for people with a dementia because of the impairments that a dementia brings and the lack of facilitation available to maintain healthy lifestyles. The reality of decision-making in most people's lives involves others who offer different perspectives and whose ideas are sought to help a relational autonomy (Jepson et al., 2016), although it is noted that this also needs further exploration when thinking about dementia (Series, 2015; Miller, Whitlatch, & Lyons, 2016). When a person develops a dementia, there may be anxiety or a lack of confidence associated with the idea that your mind can not be trusted, as described by the participants in the Safer Walking GPS Project. There may be gaps in memory or difficulties processing information, which mean that making good decisions based on sustained information may be more difficult. While the focus on the individual works to ensure that their voice is heard and their needs are met, there are others involved who are vital to achieving care (Barnes 2012), whether these are family, friends or neighbours who are concerned for their well-being. Focus on the individual can work to exclude others from the frame, and families have long felt excluded from some services such as mental health services and residential placements for people with a dementia (Brannelly, Gilmour, O'Reilly, Leighton, & Woodford, 2017). Rather than self-management, we suggest that relational care of selves points to self-care activities for the person with a dementia and their care partners. These activities are to be recognised as a need for all involved so that each can stay as well as possible through a commitment by all.

BOX 4.3 JOHN: I AM NOT READY FOR A PAID CARER TO HELP ME

John has recently had trouble arranging his clothes to use the toilet; He needs some help and this had made him rethink going to his local club, where he had been a member for some years. He commented that he would *hope to be at a competent stage* and therefore not need the help of others. John went through the routine of the meeting. He rations drinks so that he only needs to go to the toilet once at the end of the meal when everyone tends to go. Some people may be able to help him at the club, but they would need some forewarning of what was needed. An attempt at help had backfired and made things worse. During the discussion, it was clear that John could get some help to attend the club, and Fiona offered to either arrange that help or to accompany John. They agreed there were a couple of people at the club who they would ask.

Communities of care emerge through peer relationships because of shared experiences important to the person who has a dementia and their family carers. People with a dementia are supported by a complicated set of connections that are not well recognised in service provision. One way of thinking about these communities is using the Māori term whānau (pronounced far-no). A whānau is a set of people connected through experience or bonded through family and social connections. The tie may be a blood tie, where the whānau are related to each other, or it may be a set of people concerned about each other's well-being, connected by an experience or a formal grouping, having come together for a purpose. In the group are a mix of family members, friends, neighbours, peers and workers, all pulling together in solidarity to help. Some whānau or collectives of people are borne of the experience of understanding who can enable a person to be more at ease, allowing easier inclusion and participation. An acceptance of the difficulties associated with symptoms and knowledge about the experience can help people relax and share. Strong bonds are formed that are not experienced by people outside of the whānau.

Perhaps what differentiates a whānau from another community of interest is a set of values that direct actions and decisions. These are derived from Māori kaupapa and can be broadly aligned with three principles. In Māori (and other indigenous) culture(s) the collective is emphasised over the individual and has the aim of the well-being of all in the collective. Each person's prestige grows by his or her contribution to the collective good. To guide this, each person knows their responsibility – a sense of connection is central (whanaungatanga) – care is taken to ensure hospitality and kindness (manaakitanga) and guardianship is maintained to promote well-being (kaitiakitanga). These values are also present in the ethics of care (Mark, Chamberlain, & Boulton, 2017) and are consistent with relationships being central to care, requiring generosity and kindness to encourage an experience of care, with responsibility taken to make sure that care is achieved that sustains the identity and integrity of the individual and all around them.

It is suggested that an approach that recognises and values how people are faring in their experience of dementia and other coexisting conditions is adopted to replace self-management. This approach would incorporate activities that people find helpful in dealing with the everyday impacts of dementia, informed by the experiences of others who have been through similar experiences. Accepting that people with a dementia are no longer able to do certain things that they used to do is a reality of the impact of dementia and working with people to recognise that and its implications would be beneficial rather than pushing people to achieve things that are unachievable. Maintaining active decision-making falls to facilitation by others to help people with a dementia stay involved in their care. Equally important is that people who care for people with a dementia are assisted in their caring activities to enable them to sustain that for as long as possible. When care is not possible from a family carer, others may become involved to sustain a person at home.

Conclusion

Self-management is a problematic concept when applied to dementia. Instead, how people are organised to support people with a dementia in solidarity with their goals, requires a relational and caring approach dedicated to hearing the voice of experience at the centre of care but also acknowledging that everyone on the care relationship has needs that require attention. Furthermore, renewing the concept of self-management beyond this critique requires that people with a dementia contribute to that discussion, to develop an understanding that is informed by experience. In the next chapter, we turn our attention to the ethics of dementia care to examine the broad issues that are likely to arise through the progression of dementia and to examine three pertinent issues in some detail. We also present ethical frameworks to inform and guide practice.

References

Ablitt, A., Jones, G. V., & Muers, J. (2009). Living with dementia: A systematic review of the influence of relationship factors. *Ageing and Mental Health*, *13*(4), 497–511. https://doi.org/10.1080/13607860902774436

Acce, A. (2012). Type 2 diabetes and vascular dementia: Assessment and clinical strategies of care. *Advanced Practice*, *21*(6), 349–384. https://search.proquest.com/openview/801dfadce9671f2b541f45c7a21be797/1?pq-origsite=gscholar&cbl=30764

Allen, K. V., Frier, B. M., & Strachan, M. W. J. (2004). The relationship between type 2 diabetes and cognitive dysfunction: Longitudinal studies and their methodological limitations. *European Journal of Pharmacology*, *490*(1–3), 169–175. https://doi.org/10.1016/j.ejphar.2004.02.054

Barnes, M. (2012). *Care in Everyday Life*. Bristol: Policy Press.

Bodenheimer, T., Lorig, K., & Holman, H. R., Grumbach, K. (2002). Patient self-management of chronic disease in primary care. *Journal of American Medical Association*, *288*(19), 2469–2475. https://jamanetwork.com/journals/jama/article-abstract/195525?redirect=true

Boger, E., Ellis, J., Latter, S., Foster, C., Kennedy, A., Jones, F., ... Demain, S. (2015). Self-management and self-management support outcomes: A systematic review and mixed research synthesis of stakeholder views. *PLoS ONE*, *10*(7), e0130990. http://journals.plos.org/plosone/article?id=10.1371/journal.pone.0130990

Brannelly, T., Gilmour, J., O'Reilly, H., Leighton, M., & Woodford, A. (2017). An ordinary life: People with dementia living in a residential setting. *Dementia*. http://journals.sagepub.com/doi/pdf/10.1177/1471301217693169

Ellis, J., Boger, E., Latter, S., Kennedy, A., Jones, F., Foster, C., & Demain, S. (2017). Conceptualisation of the 'good' self-manager: A qualitative investigation of stakeholder views on the self-management of long-term health conditions. *Social Science & Medicine, 176*(March), 25–33. https://doi.org/10.1016/j.socscimed.2017.01.018

Feil, D., Lukman, R., Simon, B., Walston, A., & Vickery, B. (2011a). Impact of dementia on caring for patients' diabetes. *Ageing and Mental Health, 15*(7), 894–903. https://doi.org/10.1080/13607863.2011.569485

Feil, D., Rajan, M., Soroka, O., Tseng, C., Miller, D., & Pogach, L. (2011b). Risk of hypoglycaemia in older veterans with dementia and cognitive impairment: Implications for practice and policy. *JAGS, 59*(12), 2263–2272. http://onlinelibrary.wiley.com/doi/10.1111/j.1532-5415.2011.03726.x/full

Fetherstonhaugh, D., Tarzia, L., & Nay, R. (2013). Being central to decision making means I am still here!: The essence of decision making for people with dementia. *Journal of Aging Studies, 27*(2), 143–150. https://doi.org/10.1016/j.jaging.2012.12.007

Harrington, D. W., & Elliot, S. J. (2009). Weighing the importance of neighbourhood: A multilevel exploration of the determinants of overweight and obesity. *Social Science & Medicine, 68*(4), 593–600. https://doi.org/10.1016/j.socscimed.2008.11.021

Hill, J., Hicks, D., James, J., Vanterpol, G., Gillespie, C., Fox, C., & Sinclair, A. (2013). Diabetes and dementia: Guidance on practical management (October). Northampshire, UK: *Training, Research and Education for Nurses in Diabetes (TREND, UK)*, 1–24, Unpublished. https://diabetes-resources-production.s3-eu-west-1.amazonaws.com/diabetes-storage/2017-08/Diabetes_And_Dementia_Guidance_2013.pdf

Jepson, M., Laybourne, A., Williams, V., Cyhlarova, E., Williamson, T., & Robotham, D. (2016). Indirect payments: When the Mental Capacity Act interacts with the personalisation agenda. *Health and Social Care in the Community, 24*(5), 623–630. http://onlinelibrary.wiley.com/doi/10.1111/hsc.12236/full

Kirk, J. K., Arcury, T. A., Ip, E., Bell, R. A., Saldana, S., Nguyen, H. T., & Quandt, S. A. (2015). Diabetes symptoms and self-management behaviors in rural older adults. *Diabetes Research and Clinical Practice, 107*(1), 54–60. https://doi.org/10.1016/j.diabres.2014.10.005

Ledgerd, R., Hoe, J., Hoare, Z., Devine, M., Toot, S., Challis, D., & Orrell, M. (2015). Identifying the causes, prevention and management of crises in dementia. An online survey of stakeholders. *International Journal of Geriatric Psychiatry, 31*(6), 638–647. http://onlinelibrary.wiley.com/doi/10.1002/gps.4371/full

Lorig, K., & Holman, H. R. (2003). Self-management education: History, definition, outcomes, and mechanisms. *Annals of Behavioural Medicine, 26*(1), 1–7. https://doi.org/10.1207/S15324796ABM2601_01

Luchsinger, L., Palmas, W., Teresi, J., Silver, S., Kong, J., Eimicke, J., ... Shea, S. (2011). Improved diabetes control in the elderly delays global decline. *Journal of Nutrition, Health and Aging, 15*(6), 444–449. https://link.springer.com/article/10.1007/s12603-011-0057-x

Mark, G., Chamberlain, K., & Boulton, A. (2017). Acknowledging the Māori cultural values and beliefs embedded in Rongoā Māori healing. *International Journal of Indigenous Health, 12*(1), 75–92. https://search.proquest.com/openview/9857ebeb0458526da08b17ac3bc2635c/1?pq-origsite=gscholar&cbl=1356371

Miller, L. M., Whitlatch, C. J., & Lyons, K. S. (2016). Shared decision-making in dementia: A review of patient and family carer involvement. *Dementia, 15*(5), 1141–1157. http://journals.sagepub.com/doi/abs/10.1177/1471301214555542

Mountain, G. (2017). Self-management programme for people with dementia and their spouses demonstrates some benefits, but the model has limitations. *Evidence Based Nursing, 20*(1), 26–27. http://dx.doi.org/10.1136/eb-2016-102408

Nash, J. (2013). Diabetes and Wellbeing: Managing the Psychological and Emotional Challenges of Types 1 and 2. Chichester: John Wiley & Sons.

Piette, J. D., & Arbor, A. (2010). Editorial: Moving beyond the notion of 'self' care. *Chronic Illness*, 6(1), 3–6. http://journals.sagepub.com/doi/abs/10.1177/1742395309359092

Quinn, C., Anderson, D., Toms, G., Whitaker, R., Edwards, R. T., Jones, C., & Clare, L. (2014). Self-management in early-stage dementia: A pilot randomised controlled trial of the efficacy and cost-effectiveness of a self-management group intervention (The SMART study). *Trials*, 15(1), 74. https://doi.org/10.1186/1745-6215-15-74

Quinn, C., Toms, G., Jones, C., Brand, A., Edwards, R. T., Sanders, F., & Clare, L. (2016). A pilot randomized controlled trial of a self-management group intervention for people with early-stage dementia (The SMART study). *International Psychogeriatrics*, 28(5), 787–800. https://doi.org/10.1017/S1041610215002094

Ratner, E., & Atkinson, D. (2015). Why cognitive training and brain games will not prevent or forestall dementia. *Journal of the American Geriatrics Society*, 63(12), 2612–2614. http://onlinelibrary.wiley.com/doi/10.1111/jgs.1_13825/full

Scott, A. (2011). Health advocacy and self-help. In Phillips, J. (Ed.), *Te Ara—The Encylopedia of New Zealand, Social Connections: Community Organisations*. Wellington: Ministry of Culture and Heritage. http://www.teara.govt.nz/en/health-advocacy-and-self-help

Series, L. (2015). Relationships, autonomy and legal capacity: Mental capacity and support paradigms. *International Journal of Law and Psychiatry*, 40(2015), 80–91. https://doi.org/10.1016/j.ijlp.2015.04.010

Shea, S., Weinstock, R., Teresi, J., Palmas, W., Cimino, J., Lai, A., … Eimicke, J. (2009). A randomised controlled trial comparing telemedicine with usual care in older, ethnically diverse, medically underserved patients with diabetes mellitus: 5 years results of the IDEATel study. *Journal of the American Medical Information Association*, 16(4), 446–456. https://doi.org/10.1197/jamia.M3157

Sinclair, A., Girling, A., & Bayer, A. (2000). Cognitive dysfunction in older subjects with diabetes mellitus: Impact on diabetes self-management and use of care services. *Diabetes Research and Clinical Practice*, 50(3), 203–212. https://doi.org/10.1016/S0168-8227(00)00195-9

Sinclair, A., Hilison, R., & Bayer, A. (2014). Diabetes and dementia in older people: A best clinical practice statement by a multidisciplinary national expert working group. *Diabetic Medicine*, 31(9), 1024–1031. http://onlinelibrary.wiley.com/doi/10.1111/dme.12467/full

Toms, G. R., Quinn, C., Anderson, D. E., Clare, L. (2015). Help yourself: Perspectives on self-management from people with dementia and their caregivers. *Qualitative Health Research*, 25(1), 87–98. http://journals.sagepub.com/doi/abs/10.1177/10497 32314549604

University of Bradford. (2008). Bradford well-being profile. West Yorkshire, UK: *Bradford Dementia Group Division of Dementia Studies*, 1–26. https://www.bradford.ac.uk/health/media/facultyofhealthstudies/Bradford-Well-Being-Profile-with-cover-(3).pdf

Wilson, J. (2012). Evaluation of the care received by older people with diabetes. *Nursing Older People*, 24(4), 33–37. https://www.ncbi.nlm.nih.gov/pubmed/22708155

Ward, L. (2015). Caring for ourselves? Self-care and neo-liberalism. In Barnes M., Brannelly, T., Ward, L., & Ward, N. (Eds.), Ethics of Care: *Critical Advances in International Perspectives*. Bristol: Policy Press.

PART II

Towards social justice

5

ETHICS AND CARE FOR PEOPLE WITH A DEMENTIA AT HOME

Introduction

In this chapter, we provide an overview of the ethical dimensions of care at home for a person with a dementia from the literature in this field. We have selected three contested matters because they are of interest to the dementia community. For example, our discussant for this chapter, Philippa, brought to our attention the relevance and ethics of genetic testing. Philippa's thoughts are presented in the boxed text throughout the chapter. Truth telling is contested with a critical consideration of how this may impact on the relationships between people with a dementia and others, and how an acceptance of deception positions people with a dementia as passive and lacking citizenship. Difficult situations can arise whereby people with a dementia and their carers find themselves in situations where violence and aggression are present. Current responses include trying to baffle the person by hiding doors or adding locks that mean people are unable to leave or using CCTV and alarms to alert the carer when someone leaves the house. Carers are left alone to cope, often with emergency services their only backup. Finally, dementia is increasingly described as familial or hereditary. Now, open access direct to consumer predictive testing is available over the internet. Typically, consumers pay for the test kit, provide a saliva sample and a prediction is given for the likelihood of developing Alzheimer's disease, or other forms of dementia in the future. This new form of prediction operates outside of services and therefore comes without support, counter to best practice in this area. Predictive testing has been available for Fronto-temporal Lobe dementia (otherwise known as Pick's disease) and Huntington's Chorea for some time, and best practice includes a support package pre and post testing and recognition of the implications of a positive test both on the individual but also for other broader considerations, such as the availability of life insurance.

Following on from the discussions of these three topics, we turn to ethical guidance for dementia and look at the ways in which people with a dementia may remain participative. As the progress of dementia may mean that people are able to have a less direct say over their care, the ways in which their voices may be carried through the care process are explored. To build on this, we present the Nuffield ethical framework and introduce the integrity of care. Part of the ethics of care is to consider how helpful that would be to shape practices and guide interventions. The potential for transforming current approaches are discussed.

Home as a political space

Every day around the world, care occurs. It happens for children to become adults, for disabled people to live out their lives and for older people to have their needs met and it occurs, mostly, in the home. Much of the care for people with a dementia happens in their own homes, so it is no surprise that there are associated challenges to giving and receiving care. 'Good' relationships enable care, and people in care relationships need help to care well. 'Good' care requires multiple levels of help and support with skilled interventions to enable people with a dementia and their care networks to be able to care well for themselves and each other. Situations may arise where care requires difficult decisions that do not sit well with people with a dementia or carers and working out the right response requires negotiation. Care decisions may include protections that may be unwanted by people with a dementia. Therefore, home becomes a political space. How care is arranged and what resources are made available are contestable decisions, imbued with values. In this chapter, common ethical issues are presented that are relevant to life at home. Within these are the three topics we have chosen to discuss in more depth – truth telling, violence at home and genetic testing. Following this, ethical frameworks are presented to help inform decision-making to find the best possible solutions to ethical issues.

Common ethical issues in dementia

Alzheimer's Europe (2014) worked with people with a dementia and family carers to identify ethical issues throughout the course of living with a dementia. In this research, people with experience discussed how the decision to go for assessment was an ethical moment that surfaced a reality that there may be something wrong, which may not be accepted by the person being assessed. Once a diagnosis was confirmed, careful negotiations about who to disclose to and when to disclose was also pertinent. Dealing with the reactions of others prompted anxiety. Families were unsure about whether to create advance directives, how to plan proxy decision-making and when and how to implement power of attorney. Both people with a dementia and family members were aware of the balance between safety, risk and autonomy, trying to ensure that people could do as much as possible independently if it was safe and carried acceptable levels of risk to do so. Whether to tell the person with a dementia the truth, with its potential to increase distress, was identified as having no easy answer. These issues have commonality in the need for negotiation across relationships and the need for professional advice and help to find the right path.

One research project identified a comprehensive list of dementia-specific ethical issues from the perspectives of practitioners (Strech, Mertz, Knüppel, Neitzke, & Schmidhuber, 2013). As expected, these are the circumstances encountered by practitioners, which are complicated and deepened by the diverse emotional reactions of people with a dementia and their families. These are areas where practitioners feel the need to tread carefully, to avoid any potential deepening of distress in already difficult circumstances. Practitioners are cautious about how people with a dementia and their families will react and what levels of practical and emotional preparation they have about the knowledge and information they are about to encounter. Central to the ethical concerns are the uncertainties associated with diagnosis and prognosis and the limited treatments available, and therefore, being unable to provide reassurances or 'the answers' about how dementia will impact on people's lives. So here we can see that the uncertainties about diagnosis are present for both people with experience and practitioners.

Strech et al. (2013) identified that practitioners recognised that understanding and managing autonomy was delicate without a full knowledge of the person's preferences and wishes, and therefore, advanced planning was compromised. There was ambiguity in understanding competence and how best to provide information, particularly in busy clinical settings. Improvements were required in practitioner competence in assisting with best interest decision-making. Practitioners tended to underestimate the experience of carers, for example, when told by carers of the responsibilities that caring carries. In clinical settings, practitioners reported that they were not fully able to contribute to carer education and coping, for example, by exploring potential benefits and harms, or conflicts and values of their caring activities, and were therefore unable to build capacity in caregiving. Special decision-making situations such as the ability to drive, consent in sexual relationships, the suitability of genetic testing and the use of GPS (global positioning system) or other monitoring techniques raised concerns about whether the person with a dementia was adequately placed at the centre of decisions or whether others' needs were foregrounded. Likewise, these concerns arose for the prescription of antibiotics or antipsychotic drugs, covert medication giving and the use of physical restraints. End-of-life and palliative care were also identified as sites of concern. These issues reflect that professionals have anxieties about having enough information and time to make correct assessments and offer the kinds of support and therapeutic interventions that people with a dementia and their families need. More in-depth understanding of both the position of the person with a dementia and family members and their experiences would provide reassurance that the correct outcomes were decided. What the practitioners described is a lack of opportunity to delve into the complexities of care.

One key difference between practitioner identified ethical issues and those identified by people with a dementia and family members was the prospect of managing difficult care situations at home. Family carers identified this as one of the greatest challenges, whereas practitioners did not recognise its gravity in the clinic. This suggests that alternatives are required about how to decide when the care available at home is no longer sustainable and what to do about that. We reconnect with that question later in this chapter and more fully in Chapter seven on sharing responsibilities for care. In the next section, we highlight three key issues. The first is how truth telling and 'therapeutic lying' are used when memory loss causes people to request information frequently. The second is to consider responses to violence in the home towards people with a dementia and carers. Third, the support available for families who have an inherited or genetic dementia is considered, as well as the increase in availability for genetic testing that can be accessed on the internet for non-inherited dementia.

Truth telling and 'therapeutic' lying

BOX 5.1 HONESTY IS THE BEST POLICY

Phillipa described it as understandable that people do not want to upset people who can't remember. But she would prefer to be told the 'grim truth' than try to work out what is happening for herself constantly. She said, 'You need to get your head around it, and that can be difficult when the grasp slips away. It is right to ask for help and not struggle on alone and to want people to be on your side to help you.' Philippa has the greatest respect for people kicking in and doing the decent thing – helping people out when they can't remember things.

As people are more likely to talk about what is going on for them, communication is more open but that also means there are things that may be difficult to hear, articulate or deal with. People going through the experience need to discuss the grim stuff; don't blame them for wanting to discuss it. Discussion does need to happen even though the person may be devastated.

Communication is difficult when people talk to you like you are utterly brainless, unnecessary lecturing and speaking in an irritating way. Philippa described having to 'talk to yourself and give yourself a lecture that you need to just get on with it' in order to not react and tell people off for speaking to her in that way. Philippa misses [friends] when they are away, as they have a very accessible way of communicating and are supportive and friendly. They are the kind of friends you feel like you could tell anything and it would not shock them; they want to know what concerns you and they want to help you with that. Some of Phillipa's friends stepped aside and no longer visit as

---

they can't deal with it; they are a bit shocked. Close friends have remained close friends and remained helpful.

Philippa thought that sometimes it may be necessary to do things like put medication in food to make sure someone gets it if they don't understand the need for it. Asking people early on can help decide whether that may be the best thing to do.

Dementia has an impact on the ability to retain information. Being unable to retain information presents many challenges for people who experience it as lost information cannot easily be retrieved, and losses may be experienced sporadically and unpredictably. Rather than describing being unable to remember something temporarily, people with a dementia describe holes in memory, at least for a time. People develop strategies to help them remember. Not being able to retain information may lead to repetitive questioning. Others may find it difficult to answer repetitive questions, either consistently or repetitively or both. The questions may be difficult to answer as they are emotive, such as questions about diagnosis or the death of a loved one. One response that has emerged is not to tell the truth but to adopt an approach described as 'therapeutic lying' so as not to cause additional distress to people with a dementia. Recently, this issue has attracted attention because it only happens with certain groups of people, so it is apposite to ask why it is an accepted practice with people with a dementia when it would not be tolerated elsewhere.

Truth telling is essential to integrity, which is of greater moral importance to some people than others; some people may be pragmatic truth tellers whilst others are absolutist. For the former, some looseness in truth is acceptable for the right reasons, but for absolutists the truth should always be told. Depending on what positions a person takes, relationships built on honesty and integrity may be significantly harmed by lying. Where memory is impaired, people need to know they can trust people (Barnes & Brannelly, 2008), and where lying is routinely employed, this may become impossible.

Lying is described as 'endemic in dementia care settings' (Elvish, James, & Milne, 2010: 255). This questionnaire-based research identified that lying was openly accepted as a therapeutic intervention. Furthermore, presenting the results from their questionnaires at workshops with practitioners enabled the practitioners to 'hone' their deception activities so that they were justified according to the desired outcome. Seaman and Stone (2017) conducted a qualitative metasynthesis that examined deceptive practices. There was a general acceptance that deception was a therapeutic intervention when conducted in the best interests of the person and that it was usually performed to eliminate or decrease the chance of distress. The motives, modes and outcomes of deception occur in contexts that have many influencing factors, cognitive capacity being just one of them. Seaman and Stone identified that particular people deceived and that people with a dementia were understood to be incapable of deception and as such lack agency.

Most studies focus on the attitudes of paid caregivers about lying to people with a dementia and find that absolutists who would normally believe that telling the truth is always the right thing to do are persuaded that lying is therapeutic in some situations and for some reasons (Elvish et al., 2010). James (2015) considered a cognitive behavioural approach to dementia. This suggests that lying can be used to enable a connection with the person with a dementia who is 'time-shifted', and who believes that others are lying to them when in fact they are telling the truth, for example that a person has died or that their job does not exist. In this circumstance, James (ibid.) encourages lying to enter the person's experiential zone, and from there to gently rectify the time shift to orientate the person back to a place where they can understand the truth. In this situation, the use of lying is to gain trust to introduce the truth. Day, James, Meyer and Lee (2011) interviewed people living with a dementia to understand their position about being lied to as a usual aspect of care. Unsurprisingly, this group were less accepting of the need for lying as an intervention and condoned lying only in a very narrow scenario; when the person's capacity to know and understand the truth was diminished and the intervention was very much in the best interests of the person with a dementia, not for the benefit of carers or others. Even then, some of the participants with a dementia were against lying in any circumstance.

We contend that it is not the distress that is difficult to respond to but having the time to respond to the distress, especially for home care workers. More research is needed that charts the experiences of people with a dementia. Barnes and Brannelly (2008) recounted that people with a dementia are often not able to recall the name or role of the person who approaches them, so they need to trust them and use instinct to know to do so. The ability to trust someone requires a reasonable assessment that they are honest and receiving confusing responses may alert the person with a dementia to the fact that a person is unable to be honest, and therefore trustworthy.

Violence and restraint at home

> **BOX 5.2 PHILIPPA'S VIEWS ON THE TOPIC OF VIOLENCE AND RESTRAINT AT HOME**
>
> Philippa had not thought too much about this really, as it had not occurred in her experience, but thought it was a good topic to write about if it happens to people. It is a task to balance risk and personal safety and freedom. Using technology where possible can be a good answer.

Violence at home by a person with a dementia is considered a key criterion for placement in residential care. Daniel and Bowes (2011) provide a reminder that when assessing violence at home there is a need to provide distinctions between perpetrators and victims; however, these categorisations are frequently rejected by people within care relationships. In other words, the decision to accept the categorisation is a decision to admit to that violence is occurring in the knowledge that this will prompt residential placement. As this is often not wanted by either the caregiver or the person with a dementia, there is a refusal to admit violence at home. Other responses are required.

Violence is a breakdown of a care relationship and is antithetical to care. Therefore, additional support is required for the carer and person with a dementia. It is essential to note that people with a dementia may face violence from others. Kishimoto et al. (2013) surveyed family carers in Japan who care for people with mild cognitive impairment and 15% reported shouting or screaming at the person with a dementia or threatening abandonment or placement in a home. These findings are broadly consistent elsewhere (Wiglesworth et al., 2010). VandeWeerd, Paveza, Walsh and Corvin (2013) suggest that professionals adopt a risk profile approach that considers aspects such as low self-esteem and alcohol misuse of carers, alongside the propensity for aggression from people with a dementia to assess the likelihood of violence. Killick, Taylor, Begley, Carter Anand and O'Brien's (2015) systematic review of the literature identified that there was very limited evidence from the perspective of people with a dementia about what constituted abuse.

Living at home with a dementia often carries a balance of independence, risk and freedom in the face of increased dependency. Meanwhile, well-meaning but under-resourced responses available to people living with people with a dementia may mean that there are micro injustices such as limitations placed on the ability to go out (Bartlett, 2016). In Brannelly's (2004) research, a mental health nurse participant whose father had a dementia commented that she had finally lost her patience with him in the middle of the night as he repeatedly tried to leave the house. She was staying with him to give her mum a break, as this had been a nightly recurrence for a couple of weeks and her mum was exhausted. She recounted that she had shouted at him, and he became very upset and angry with her. It did not improve the situation and she felt terrible that her training and skills were lost in that moment. But mostly it made the mental health nurse reflect that professional caregivers go home at the end of their working day and do not give much thought to the many carers in this situation.

Carers may discuss elements of challenging behaviours such as verbal and physical aggression at home. Some carers may implement strategies to avoid violence, or may be living with violence because they have no help available to them. Some may see an admission of violence as an indicator of not being able to sustain their caring role and therefore raise the possibility of residential care. The fear of placement in residential care is suspecting that the well-being of the person with a dementia would be further deteriorated (we do note that it may not be realistic but it is still feared). If we consider the levels of aggression in care homes, then it is apparent that moving a person with a dementia who is violent towards caregivers moves the issue to another place for the person to be violent towards other caregivers. It would seem that strategies for dealing with the aggression are not as forthcoming as they may be for other groups. What interventions are currently available to help people decrease frustration and thereby deal with aggression?

Mostly, responses to help people reduce aggression can be described as *soft paternalism* (Smebye, Kirkevold, & Enderdal, 2016), that is strategies that aim to prevent poor decisions resulting in poorer outcomes for the person with a dementia. Smebye et al. (2016) recommend that soft paternalism is acceptable if the decisions reflect a longer-term aim for care, such as the person with a dementia remaining at home. Interventions at present include activities during the day to promote better sleep and decrease nighttime waking, covering exits to disguise them, removing keys and access to the outdoors at night, using baffle locks or other ways of decreasing the ability of the person with a dementia to be able to open doors and installing technologies such as alerts and CCTV. Depending on the person with a dementia, some of these are likely to increase frustration rather than allay it, and their response to them should guide a review of them. We suggest that the approach taken and the reasons for it are discussed with the person with a dementia and that the longer-term aim is explicitly recorded. In our experience, these approaches are likely to work for a time and then adaptations and new approaches will be required. We also need to add new ways of helping people with a dementia stay at home, which would be best designed by people facing the experience – people with a dementia themselves.

Genetic testing for dementia – ethical issues

BOX 5.3 GENETIC TESTING AND PICK'S DISEASE. 'IT'S SO FRIGHTENING WHEN YOU THINK THIS IS GOING TO BE ME'

Philippa lost three of her five siblings and her mother to Pick's disease and now has it herself. She looked after her mum, so there are no secrets about what is coming. She is grateful that times have changed, as people used to be locked away in their home, out of sight, and it is more accepted now. Phillipa welcomes social movements like the Alzheimer's Society on the High Street so many places, as that helps it be visible and not hidden away. It is a sign of how times have changed. It is important to have informal advertising where people with a dementia educate others about the disease and what it is like to have it.

Pick's disease is an inherited form of early-onset dementia. Phillipa says it is terrible to see your siblings die from the disease. One brother who Philippa described as a giant personality experienced physical and psychological deterioration. Another brother lived in Canada and was looked after by a friend. Philippa regretted not being able to get to his funeral. She learnt a lot from those losses, seeing such a great big personality shrink.

> Philippa, her children and her sister are participants in a research study in London. They attend every year to be scanned and tested. Her children have had the genetic test for Pick's disease and know whether they will develop it or not. Philippa described her son and daughter as the bravest people she knows, as it is really tricky knowing what is ahead. She had never been offered genetic testing as it was not available at the time and so lived in fear of whether she would develop it or not. She would have liked an answer, but potentially not the implications of the answer. Philippa's son and daughter were offered support before, during and after the test and counselling. There was nothing else that could have been done better. The family members are fully supportive of contributing to research and looking for a cure or treatment for Pick's disease.

Recent rapid advances in genetic testing for neurodegenerative diseases have resulted in increased susceptibility testing for 'at-risk' individuals, and a new era of genetic discovery is beckoning (Po et al., 2014). Direct to consumer predictability testing is available on the internet, but the question is who benefits from this and whether there is a responsibility to provide support to people who access predictability testing. Clear clinical indication for the need for genetic testing occurs when a detailed family history identifies strong familial links, particularly for early-onset dementias (Roberts & Uhlmann, 2013). Loy, Schofield, Turner and Kwok (2014) suggest that a significant family history includes many affected members over consecutive generations. Of the dementias, Frontotemporal dementia (FTD), also known as Pick's disease, is hereditary. A hereditary incidence occurs in about 60% of people diagnosed with FTD, of whom 20% have an identified genetic cause, which leaves a definitive cause for FTD unknown (Po et al., 2014). Alzheimer's disease has a less strong hereditary association and having a family history does not mean there is a genetic cause or mendelian factor. A mendelian or single gene disease has a genetic mutation of a single gene known to cause a disease. In dementia, these are very rare, and most incidences are a complex interaction of environmental and genetic factors. Thus, most people with a family history of dementia do not need genetic predictability testing (Loy et al., 2014: 828).

The blueprint for neurodegenerative genetic tests started with Huntington's disease (or Chorea) in the 1970s (Arribas-Ayllon, 2011). Roberts and Uhlmann (2013) identified that test access, informed consent, risk estimation and communication, the return of results and policies to prevent genetic discrimination all presented ethical issues in practice. Huntington's disease is predicted by a sensitive genetic test that is 99% correct, couched in three test meetings. A pre-test meeting has psychotherapeutic assessment, the second gains consent and conducts the test and the third discloses the test result. A support person is encouraged to attend, and the test is available to adults only (Roberts & Uhlmann, 2013). This is the gold standard of genetic testing designed to work alongside the person to understand their experience and interpretation of the test, to answer questions that they may have about what the information means for them and their family's future and any obligations they may have, for example, those that affect life insurance. Farsides (2011) acknowledged that the choice to have the test moves people from a categorisation of at risk, to (pre)symptomatic.

Apolipoprotein E (APOE) testing for Alzheimer's disease has largely been discouraged because the limitation of the accuracy of testing means that predictability is low. The affected gene may be present, but the disease may not develop. It is widely accepted that there is a familial form with autosomal dominant inheritance in Alzheimer's disease, Parkinson's disease and other prion-based diseases, but that this accounts for a minority of cases. Despite this, direct to consumer (DTC) testing is available for people who are concerned about the possibility of developing a disease that is present in their family. In the UK, for example, tests cost approximately £150–250 and require a saliva sample to be posted to the test facility and returned with a list of genetic susceptibilities, including those for Alzheimer's disease, other neurological diseases and other physical health conditions (see, for example, Alzheimer's Society website https://www.alzheimers.org.uk/info/20008/symptoms_and_diagnosis). In contrast to the gold standard, in DTC tests no support is provided. Roberts and Uhlmann (2013) argue strongly that clinical services are best placed to host genetic testing because of the complexities of interpretation and the sensitivities of disclosure.

A review of 41 studies about the quality of life (Paulsen et al., 2013) after predictive neurogenetic testing found that, despite concerns over increased testing, people were resilient on disclosure, and that overall, increased testing would advance clinical care. Paulsen et al. (2013: 2) identified that catastrophic outcomes are rare, increased anxiety and depression was transient; participants mostly did not regret the test and reported the benefits of knowing. Currently, discrimination based on test results is poorly understood and requires more policy and research to inform practice; for example, Fulda and Lykens (2006) recognised the implications of the results of positive genetic testing for employment and insurance purposes.

While there is more research available about experiences of genetic testing in Huntington's disease, the issues for other dementias are more obscure given the uncertainty between testing positive and developing the disease. In one qualitative study of the experiences of adult children of parents with young-onset dementia (Aslett, Huws, Woods, & Kelly Rhind, 2017), participants reflected on their experiences of living with the prospect of the increased likelihood of developing a dementia at a young age. One of the five participants had been offered genetic counselling and decided not to proceed with testing as the counsellor noted that if she tested positive she would need to consider not having children. This was untenable to the participant as she realised if her parent had been offered the same advice she would not have been born. As diagnostic testing becomes more prevalent, more evidence will be available about the experiences of living with the chances of transmitting a hereditary disease and how people make decisions about testing and disclosure within families.

Summary

The thread that runs through these ethical issues is that dementia presents situations where there are opportunities to care well. A disconnect with reality or difficulty answering 'grim' questions may press people into shortcuts that avoid the truth, which may disrupt trust and solidarity. Violence may be a reaction to being confined in one place or at home, not being able to find the door or finding doors locked. More resources need to be available rather than leaving families to face violence alone. For some families, the prospect of genetic or hereditary dementia looms over the future – a terrifying notion as Philippa describes. Any testing for dementia requires sensitive and careful work to enable people to understand the implications of it and what it means for the future. Next, we turn our attention to the Nuffield ethical framework and return to the ethics of care to consider how to guide good practice with people with a dementia.

Guiding care with ethical approaches

Ethical frameworks are needed that recognise that people with a dementia can participate when facilitated to do so and that the responsibility for participation remains with others to make it happen. The most useful dementia specific ethical framework is the *Nuffield Council on Bioethics, Dementia: Ethical issues* (2009). Building ethical responses to people with a dementia is shaped by many factors, which take into account the experiences of having a dementia and caring for the person. This includes the resources available, the knowledge and skills of people providing support and what is known about the experience of dementia. The Nuffield Council (2009: 20) ethics guide is a six-component framework to improve ethical decision-making for people working with people with a dementia and others, including family members. They suggest:

1. A care-based approach to ethical decisions. Ethical decisions can be approached in a three-stage process: (a) identifying the relevant facts; (b) interpreting and applying appropriate ethical values to those facts and (c) comparing the situation with other similar situations to find ethically relevant similarities or differences.
2. A belief about the nature of dementia. Dementia arises as a result of a brain disorder and is harmful to the individual.
3. A belief about the quality of life with a dementia. With good care and support, people with a dementia can expect to have a good quality of life throughout the course of their illness.
4. The importance of promoting the interests of both the person with a dementia and those who care for them. People with a dementia have interests, both in

their autonomy and their well-being. Promoting autonomy involves enabling and fostering relationships that are important to the person and supporting them in maintaining their sense of self and expressing their values. Autonomy is not simply to be equated with the ability to make rational decisions. A person's well-being includes both their moment-to-moment experiences of contentment or pleasure and more objective factors such as their level of cognitive functioning. The separate interests of carers must be recognised and promoted.

5. The requirement to act in accordance with solidarity. The need to recognise the citizenship of people with a dementia, and to acknowledge mutual interdependence and responsibility to support people with a dementia both within families and in society as a whole.

6. Recognising personhood, identity and value. The person with a dementia remains the same, equally valued person throughout the course of their illness, regardless of the extent of the changes in their cognitive and other functions.

This framework clearly places care and interdependence at the centre of ethical practice for people with a dementia. As we introduced in Chapter one, care and interdependence are central to the ethics of care. Attentiveness also features, so that the needs of family carers are considered alongside those of people with a dementia. Avoiding blame and reacting to people with a dementia in a way that acknowledges their behaviour as part of their illness is also valued. Solidarity with people with a dementia is also supported. In addition to these useful points, the ethics of care asks about fairness and equality for people with a dementia, therefore, identifying and taking responsibility to help people with a dementia who face inequality to become more equal.

In Chapter one we introduced the key aspects of the ethics of care, that include interdependence, recognising marginalisation and promoting equality, and here we return to another prong of the ethics of care – the integrity of care. Tronto (1993; 2013) developed the integrity of care to critique and guide caring practices. According to Tronto (2013), caring includes:

- *Caring about – attentiveness*: At this first phase of care, someone or some group notices unmet caring needs. If attentiveness is not present, then the other elements of care ethics cannot be practiced. Openness, recognition, respect for identity and diversity are required. In care situations, the needs of all are noted, and the course of action taken can be measured against these to understand whose needs have been met.

- *Caring for – responsibility*: Once needs are identified, someone or some group has to take responsibility to make certain that these needs are met. Assuming responsibility to act on the basis of the needs identified in attentiveness requires 'judging with care', applying the ethics of care to the process to consider the direction care takes and what outcomes are likely. Attempting to meet, but not actually meeting needs indicates a failure of responsibility.

The Mental Capacity Act (MCA, 2005) intends to empower people with a dementia and others who have long-term incapacity to make specific and timely decisions regarding their own care, the freedom to choose, self-determine and take risks. It also provides protections for those making proxy decisions by encouraging engagement with the preferences of people with a dementia to find creative solutions that meet needs.

For many people with a dementia and their families, making decisions about care are usual occurrences of daily life, if complicated by the addition of conditions such as dementia. The progressive illness promises future disablement and increasing needs as families figure how best to accommodate this (Barnes, 2012), with the expectation of help from services when needed. Practitioners are more knowledgeable and comfortable approaching discussions about financial management and power of attorney but less so for more complex issues (Manthorpe, Samsi, & Rapaport, 2014), even in acute hospital settings where decisions about place loom large, leaving people with a dementia and families unprepared for these discussions (Poole et al., 2014).

Family members faced with proxy decision-making are left unsupported by practitioners (Livingstone et al., 2010) and found that decision-making is more difficult where the decision goes against the wishes of the person with a dementia (Manthorpe et al., 2014). Because there is an expectation that care home placement is an inevitability in many places for people with a dementia, this sets a tone for the discussions that may be had about staying at home. Figure 5.1 shows how decision-making capacity can be assessed.

In many countries, for example Australia, best interest decisions are made on an ad hoc basis (Purser, Magner, & Madison, 2015). In England and Wales, the Mental Capacity Act (MCA) was introduced as a national standard that provides protections for those making proxy decisions by encouraging engagement with the preferences of people with a dementia to find creative solutions that meet their needs. The five guiding principles of the MCA are (1) assume capacity; (2) take all practicable steps to help the person make the decision; (3) people may make unwise decisions; (4) anything done for the person must

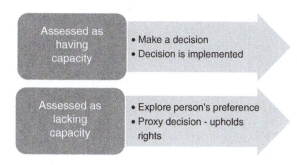

FIGURE 5.1   Assessing capacity

be in their best interests and (5) take the least restrictive action to preserve rights and freedom.

Described as having the power to transform the lives of many (House of Lords, 2014), the MCA has yet to achieve that vision. In the UK, despite the introduction of the MCA, capacity assessment remains the domain of specialists rather than generalist practice (Jayes, Palmer, & Enderby, 2016; Marshall & Sprung, 2016; Murrell & McCalla, 2016). Capacity is still questioned when the person's choice is incongruent with the consensus of others (Poole et al., 2014), or carries risks intolerable to others. Furthermore, a person may be assessed as lacking capacity because they do not understand the consequences of their decision, such as wanting to return home with help, but the level of help they require is not available (Cliff & McGraw, 2016).

Conclusion

People with a dementia appreciate the acknowledgement and recognition that comes with being involved, but are not always offered that opportunity (Fetherstonhaugh, Tarzia, & Nay, 2016). Hedman, Hansebo, Ternestedt, Hellstrom and Norberg (2012) noted that people with a dementia experienced offensive behaviours from others, such as an assumption of absolute incapability to understand anything, and tried to help people understand they were able to understand and respond. Brannelly (2011) identified that some practitioners assumed an inability to participate that was based on social regard for the person with a dementia. It remains the responsibility of those around people with a dementia to ensure that everything possible is done to continue their contribution to life.

References

Alzheimer's Europe. (2014). *Ethical Dilemmas Faced by Carers and People with Dementia.* Luxembourg: Alzheimer's Europe.

Arribas-Ayllon, M. (2011). The ethics of disclosing genetic diagnosis for Alzheimer's disease: Do we need a new paradigm? *British Medical Bulletin, 100*(1), 7–21. https://www.researchgate.net/profile/Michael_Arribas-Ayllon/publication/51218965_The_ethics_of_disclosing_genetic_diagnosis_for_Alzheimers_disease_Do_we_need_a_new_paradigm/links/56eaacde08ae8c97677b9082.pdf

Aslett, H. J., Huws, J. C., Woods, R. T., & Kelly-Rhind, J. (2017). 'This is killing me inside': The impact of having a parent with young-onset dementia. *Dementia.* https://doi.org/10.1177/1471301217702977

Barnes, M. (2012). *Care in Everyday Life.* Bristol: Policy Press.

Barnes, M., & Brannelly, T. (2008). Achieving care and social justice for people with dementia. *Nursing Ethics, 15*(3), 384.

Bartlett, R. (2016). Scanning the conceptual horizons of citizenship. *Dementia, 15*(3), 453–461. http://journals.sagepub.com/doi/abs/10.1177/1471301216644114

Bourgault, S. (2016). Attentive listening and care in a neoliberal era: Weilian insights for hurried times. *Ethics and Politics, XVIII*(3), 311–377. http://www2.units.it/etica/2016_3/BOURGAULT.pdf

Brannelly, P. M. (2004). *Citizenship and care for people with dementia*. Unpublished PhD Thesis. University of Birmingham.

Brannelly, T. (2011). Sustaining citizenship: Older people with dementia and the phenomenon of social death. *Nursing Ethics, 18*(5), 662–671. http://journals.sagepub.com/doi/abs/10.1177/0969733011408049

Cliff, C., & McGraw, C. (2016). The conduct and process of mental capacity assessments in home health care settings. *British Journal of Community Nursing, 21*(11), 570–577. https://doi.org/10.12968/bjcn.2016.21.11.570

Daniel, B., & Bowes, A. (2011). Re-thinking harm and abuse: Insights from a lifespan perspective. *British Journal of Social Work, 41*(5), 820–836. https://doi.org/10.1093/bjsw/bcq116

Day, A. M., James, I. A., Meyer, T. D., & Lee, D. R. (2011). Do people with dementia find lies and deception in dementia care acceptable? *Aging & Mental Health, 15*(7), 822–829. https://doi.org/10.1080/13607863.2011.569489

Elvish, R., James, I., & Milne, D. (2010). Lying in dementia care: An example of a culture that deceives in people's best interests. *Aging & Mental Health, 14*(3), 255–262. https://doi.org/10.1080/13607861003587610

Farsides, B. (2011). Courage, compassion and communication: Young people and Huntington's disease. *Clinical Ethics, 6*(2), 55. http://journals.sagepub.com/doi/full/10.1258/ce.2011.011022

Fetherstonhaugh, D., Tarzia, L., & Nay, R. (2016). Being central to decision making means I am still here!: The essence of decision making for people with dementia, *Journal of Aging Studies, 27*(2), 143–150. https://doi.org/10.1016/j.jaging.2012.12.007

Fulda, K. G., & Lykens, K. (2006). Ethical issues in predictive genetic testing: A public health perspective, *Journal of Medical Ethics, 32*(2), 143–147. http://jme.bmj.com/content/32/3/143.short

Hedman, R., Hansebo, G., Ternestedt, B. M., Hellstrom, I., & Norberg, A. (2012). How people with Alzheimer's disease express their sense of self: Analysis using Rom Harre's theory of selfhood. *Dementia, 12*(6), 713–733. http://journals.sagepub.com/doi/abs/10.1177/1471301212444053

House of Lords (2014). *Mental Capacity Act 2005: Post-Legislative Scrutiny*, House of Lords, London.

James, I. A. (2015). The use of CBT in dementia care: A rationale for Communication and Interaction Therapy (CAIT) and therapeutic lies. *The Cognitive Behaviour Therapist, 8*(e10), 1. https://doi.org/10.1017/S1754470X15000185

Jayes, M., Palmer, R., & Enderby, P. (2016). An exploration of mental capacity assessment within acute hospital and intermediate care settings in England: A focus group study. *Disability and Rehabilitation, 39*(21), 2148–2157. https://doi.org/10.1080/09638288.2016.1224275

Killick, C., Taylor, B. J., Begley, E., Carter Anand, J., & O'Brien, M. (2015). Older people's conceptualization of abuse: A systematic review, *Journal of Elder Abuse & Neglect, 27*(2), 100–120. https://doi.org/10.1080/08946566.2014.997374

Kishimoto, Y., Terada, S., Takeda, N., Oshima, E, Honda, H., Yoshida H., … Uchitomi, Y. (2013). Abuse of people with cognitive impairment by family caregivers in Japan (a cross-sectional study). *Psychiatry Research, 209*(3), 699–704. https://doi.org/10.1016/j.psychres.2013.01.025

Livingstone, G., Leavey, G., Manela, M., Livingston, D., Rait, G., Sampson E., … Cooper C. (2010). Making decisions for people with dementia who lack capacity: Qualitative study of family carers in UK. *British Medical Journal, 341*(c4184). https://doi.org/10.1136/bmj.c4184

Loy, C. L., Schofield, P. R., Turner, A. M., & Kwok, J. B. J. (2014). Genetics of dementia. *Lancet, 383*(9919), 828–840. http://dx.doi.org/10.1016/S0140-6736(13)60630-3

Manthorpe, J., Samsi, K., & Rapaport, J. (2014). Dementia nurses' experience of the Mental Capacity Act 2005: A follow up study. *Dementia, 13*(1), 131–143. http://journals.sagepub.com/doi/abs/10.1177/1471301212454354

Marshall, H., & Sprung, S. (2016). The Mental Capacity Act: A review of the current literature. *British Journal of Community Nursing, 21*(8), 406–410. https://doi.org/10.12968/bjcn.2016.21.8.406

Mental Capacity Act (MCA). (2005). *Mental Capacity Act 2005*. London: Department of Health, Stationary Office.

Murrell, A., & McCalla, L. (2016). Assessing decision-making capacity: The interpretation and implementation of the Mental Capacity Act 2005 amongst social care professionals. *Practice, 28*(1), 21–36. https://doi.org/10.1080/09503153.2015.1074667

Nuffield Council on Bioethics (2009). *Dementia: Ethical Issues*. London: Nuffield Council on Bioethics.

Paulsen, J. S., Nance, M., Kim, J. I., Carlozzi N. E., Panegyres P. K., Erwin C., … Williams, J. K. (2013). A review of quality of life after predictive testing for and earlier identification of neurodegenerative diseases. *Progress in Neurobiology, 110*(November), 2–28. http://dx.doi.org/10.1016/j.pneurobio.2013.08.003

Po, K., Leslie, F. V. C., Gracia, N., Bartley, L., Kwok, J. B. J., Halliday G. M., … Burrell, J. R. (2014). Heritability in frontotemporal dementia: More missing pieces? *Journal of Neurology, 261*(11), 2170–2177. https://link.springer.com/article/10.1007/s00415-014-7474-9

Poole, M., Bond, J., Emmett, C., Greener, H., Louw, S. J., Robinson, L., & Hughes, J. C. (2014). Going home? An ethnographic study of assessment of capacity and best interests in people with dementia being discharged from hospital. *BMC Geriatrics, 14*(1), 56. https://doi.org/10.1186/1471-2318-14-56

Purser, K., Magner, E. S., & Madison J. (2015). A therapeutic approach to assessing legal capacity in Australia. *International Journal of Law and Psychiatry, 38*(January–February), 18–28. https://doi.org/10.1016/j.ijlp.2015.01.003

Roberts, S. J., & Uhlmann, W. R. (2013). Genetic susceptibility testing for neurodegenerative diseases: Ethical and practice issues. *Progress in Neurobiology, 110*(November), 89–101. https://doi.org/10.1016/j.pneurobio.2013.02.005

Seaman, A. T., & Stone, A. M. (2017). Little white lies, interrogating the (un)acceptability of deception in the context of dementia. *Qualitative Health Research, 27*(1), 60–76. http://journals.sagepub.com/doi/10.1177/1049732315618370

Smebye, K. L., Kirkevold, M., & Engedal, K. (2016). Ethical dilemmas concerning autonomy when persons with dementia wish to live at home: A qualitative, hermeneutic study. *BMC Health Services Research, 16*(1), 21. https://doi.org/10.1186/s12913-015-1217-1

Strech, D., Mertz, M., Knüppel, H., Neitzke, G., & Schmidhuber, M. (2013). The full spectrum of ethical issues in dementia care: Systematic qualitative review. *The British Journal of Psychiatry, 202*(6), 400–406. https://www.ncbi.nlm.nih.gov/pubmed/23732935

Tronto, J. C. (1993). *Moral Boundaries: A Political Argument for an Ethic of Care*. New York: New York University Press.

Tronto, J. C. (2013). *Caring Democracy*. New York: New York University Press.

Tuckett, A. G. (2012). The experience of lying in dementia care: A qualitative study, *Nursing Ethics, 19*(1), 7–20. https://www.ncbi.nlm.nih.gov/pubmed/22140189

VandeWeerd, C., Paveza, G. J., Walsh, M., & Corvin, J. (2013). Physical mistreatment in persons with Alzheimer's disease. *Journal of Aging Research*, Article ID 920324, 1–10. http://dx.doi.org/10.1155/2013/920324

Wiglesworth, A., Mosqueda, L., Mulnard, R., Liao, S., Gibbs, L., & Fitzgerald, W. (2010). Screening for abuse and neglect of people with dementia. *Journal of the American Geriatrics Society*, *58*(3), 493–500. http://onlinelibrary.wiley.com/doi/10.1111/j.1532-5415.2010.02737.x/full

6

TECHNOLOGICAL ENHANCED CARE AND CITIZENSHIP

Introduction

Life at home for people with a dementia inevitably involves technologies. These include household appliances like remote controls and ovens, as well as doors, locks, switches, telephones and lighting. Technologies like these are shaping people's lives every single day; they have become so assimilated into our lifestyles and homes that we may not even think of them as technologies – but of course, they are. A technology is anything derived from scientific knowledge. Some technologies are integral to a person's health and well-being, including items such as dentures, spectacles, and hearing and mobility aids. Such items become an extension of the person and are therefore important to consider in the context of technological care and citizenship. Modern forms of communication technology can enhance a person's agentic capacity. For example, voice recognition software, which is a common feature on most modern tablets and smartphones (e.g. Siri, Google Now and Cortana), responds to requests for information. In this chapter, we foreground the relationships people have with everyday technologies, particularly digital technologies, and consider how everyday technologies of today and the future have the potential to transform the meaning and nature of care and citizenship at home.

Arguably, there has been a degree of technophobia within dementia studies. Most research and practice guidance focus on human relationships rather than the relationships people have with technologies. The 'Triangle of Care' model, for example, which describes a therapeutic relationship between the person with a dementia, staff member and carer, does not refer to technologies at all (Hannan, Thompson, Worthington, & Rooney, 2013). Yet our relationships with technologies are as embedded in everyday life as our relationships with other people. Reflect for a moment on how often you check your Smartphone or use the internet, even when you are with other people. Consider, as well, how many people with a dementia say they have trouble getting dressed, taking medications and using pill dispensers, and dealing with money. Clearly, technologies are a 'complicating aspect' of life at home (Malinowsky, Almkvist, Kottorp, & Nygård, 2010: 2). Thus, we regard technologies in terms of another relational element in a person's life and marshal the idea of 'technological citizenship' to ask questions about whether our rights and obligations as citizens should change as technology changes (Frankenfield, 1992).

When the use of technology by people with a dementia is addressed, the emphasis has been on technological interventions and the potential risks of trying to do things *to* people rather than with them (see, for example, Astell, 2006). More recent studies have begun to focus instead on the usability of gadgets designed to support basic care and household tasks (i.e. assistive technologies) such as memory aids and key fobs (e.g. Gibson, Dickinson, Brittain, & Robinson, 2015). Our concern in this chapter is primarily with the relationships people have with everyday technologies and the support that individuals and families are likely to need to access and use them (rather than the technologies themselves).

Technologies are often perceived of as 'cold' in comparison to 'warm' care, although it is questionable whether or not this is a meaningful opposition (Pols & Moser, 2009). The reality often is that everyday technologies can enhance care and citizenship, given the right mindset and support. In our view, people with a dementia need relational support that is technical, as well as emotional. We define technological relational support as practical assistance with everyday technologies such as clothing, mobility aids, medication and digital devices, and caring about a person's access to and use of everyday technologies. It can involve basic things such as laying clothes out on beds, ensuring the person has the right amount of money and helping someone to (re) use computer equipment. Alternatively, technological relational support can involve more sophisticated activities, such as checking a person's medications (Fiss et al., 2013) or overseeing a person's social media activities in the face of declining decision-making capacity (Batchelor, Bobrowicz, Mackenzie, & Milne, 2012). Research suggests that people with a dementia who live alone are likely to find it particularly challenging to cope with technology (Evans, Price, & Meyer, 2016). Hence, this group may be most in need of technological relational support. The question of whose responsibility it is to provide such support is discussed in the next chapter, our focus here is on explaining the notion of technological care and citizenship for people with a dementia living at home.

Technological relational support begins by foregrounding the care needs and rights of the person with a dementia. There is a tendency within dementia studies to prioritise the perspective of the caregiver rather than the person with a dementia, especially when it comes to evaluating the benefits of a new technology. For example, most of what we know about the use of GPS enabled 'location' technologies is based on information elicited from family carers and/or clinicians rather than people with a dementia. Whilst caregivers offer an important perspective, so too can people with a dementia when given the right opportunity to share their experiences. From a disability rights perspective, it is imperative that we find out about and seek to overcome the challenges facing someone with a dementia when trying to access and use everyday technologies. This is what technological care and citizenship are all about.

As part of the preparation for this chapter, Bartlett spoke to a married couple in their late 50s about their use of everyday technologies and views on the proposed content of this chapter. Box 6.1 contains a summary of the conversation.

BOX 6.1 INTRODUCING KAREN AND MARTIN AND THEIR VIEWS ON TECHNOLOGY

Karen and Martin are a married couple in their late 50s. Karen was diagnosed with Alzheimer's disease when she was 55 years old. She used to work in a bank and used computers and the internet on a daily basis. Martin recently retired and sees himself as Karen's full-time carer. Ahead of my visit, I sent an email to Martin and Karen containing a 200-word summary of the chapter, which included a link to the Dem@Care study video.

On introducing the topic of technologies at the start of my visit, Karen laughed and said 'next', suggesting it was a topic that she would rather not think about. Nevertheless, during the conversation, Karen told me that she had asked for a new tablet for Christmas because she wanted to try to use one again. Martin spoke of the benefits of being able to do online shopping, thus avoiding the shops, which he said Karen found 'too much'.

Speaking to Karen and Martin led to a rethink on focusing entirely on digital technologies, as Karen mentioned clothing and Martin said how Karen leaves lights on. This is significant because it shows how everyday technologies can affect a person's life and interactions with others. Karen had asked for a tablet device for Christmas as she wants to try to use it. The cost of digital equipment was a concern, especially the monitoring devices. For Karen, owning and using a tablet again seemed to be about feeling accomplished with technology rather than technology being integrated into her life because of her dementia. I asked them what they thought of the Dem@Care study video. Martin had watched it and questioned the affordability of such systems.

The chapter is organised into three parts; the first part introduces the idea of technological care and citizenship by outlining the relational context before recounting two real-life stories of various technologies being used to enable a person with a dementia to live at home. This sets the scene for a detailed discussion in the second part about using everyday technologies to enhance care, and in the third part it is about using everyday technologies to enhance citizenship. We realise that this distinction is somewhat problematic (as care and citizenship are often intertwined), but we use it to clarify the distinct potentials of everyday technologies.

Everyday life, everyday (digital) technologies

People with a dementia are surrounded by technologies (as we all are) designed to make life easier, but which can also make it frustrating. Modern technologies are often invisible, which can be both helpful and unhelpful. For example, many public toilets and washrooms now have sensor taps, which are great once you know where the sensor activator pad is, but until then you can be waving your hands around everywhere. Similarly, Wi-Fi within the home allows devices and sound systems to connect automatically with each other. This feels lovely to use when they are working but annoying when they break down. To improve life at home for people with a dementia, we need to acknowledge the micro-frustrations and 'joys' that everyday technologies can bring into people's lives. In particular, we need to examine the extent to which everyday technologies are making possible or hindering a liveable life at home for people with a dementia.

As we mentioned in Chapter three, one area where there has been considerable research is memory aids. In recent years, this has expanded to electronic memory aids, which include a range of devices designed to support memory, including electronic calendars and clocks, as well as digital apps. For example, one small-scale intervention study conducted recently aimed to examine the use of MindMate – a specifically designed memory app for people with a dementia, downloadable from iTunes (McGoldrick, 2017). The work was based on a sample of three participants (two men and one woman), all of whom had a diagnosis of (mild) Alzheimer's disease and were living at home. Participants were asked to identify events they wanted to remember (such as attend doctor's appointment, phone a relative, make something to eat) and when they wanted to be reminded of them. The app was then set up to remind people of these events using an alarm. As the author points out, participants needed technical support to use the app, which she was able to provide, but they found it useful. However, even in this small-scale study, one participant dropped out because she found the alarm sound 'annoying' and according to her partner, she was struggling to use her smartphone generally (p. 42). Additionally, there were several bugs with the app, which would have hampered people's experience of using it.

Relationships with technologies are often tangible and visible, meaning they have the capacity to reveal things. Using or not attempting to use a technology can show how well a person is coping with the experience of a dementia – as we saw in the example given above. Similarly, you might recall how William (who we met in Chapter two) would mistake his TV remote control for a telephone, and so he would pick that up when he heard the phone ring and miss calls. This scenario shows how even the most basic forms of technology can place significant demands on an older person with a dementia and frailty.

When everyday technologies break down or go wrong, it can be challenging for a person with a dementia to work out what to do. This is especially true for people with a dementia who live alone. For example, one community-based worker recalls phoning a client to remind her about attending day care, but the client said, 'I can't come today. Well my house is full of water, there's water everywhere, I don't know where it's coming from.' As the researchers explain, 'the community care professional was able to organize immediate assistance to manage the leaking toilet', but the person with dementia lacked the capacity to be able to respond appropriately to the unexpected problem (Evans et al., 2016: 8). This show how any disruption to the smooth running of an everyday technology (i.e. plumbing) can be destabilising and a threat to living well at home if no one is alerted to the problem.

Because our relationships with technologies (or lack of) are visible, they can reveal a person's vulnerabilities. This may be why some people with a dementia are hesitant about using certain kinds of technology. For example, younger, physically fit people with early-onset dementia may be reluctant to use any kind of technology that says 'I am vulnerable' – like a 'falls' pendant or walking stick. Alternatively, others may be proud of the fact that they have a technology to support them – as was the case with some of the people with a dementia who took part in the Safer Walking GPS Project. Such divergences show how important it is to conceive of vulnerability positively as 'openness', as opposed to only negatively as 'weakness' (Wiles, 2011: 573). Moreover, they remind us of the need to consider everyday technologies according to their 'usefulness for people with mild cognitive impairment (MCI) and early stages of dementia on the one hand, and people with moderate or severe dementia on the other' (Rosenberg, Kottorp, & Nygård, 2012: 5). This is particularly important given the growing expectation that citizens will use (or at least accept) digital technologies into their lives to look after themselves and each other.

Digital technologies are seen as the future for supporting the delivery of health care in many parts of the world, including England (NHS England, 2014) and Denmark (The Danish Government, 2013). The belief is that 'with digital welfare services, it is possible to make everyday life easier for citizens – at less cost' (The Danish Government, 2013: 3). Before we consider this proposition in relation to people with a dementia at home, it is important to clarify what is meant by digital technologies. Digital technologies are devices that transmit codes and signals between different devices and allow immense amounts of information to be stored and transmitted. One way of showing the distinction between a low-tech and digital technology is by looking at what one French walking stick maker is doing with its products. The company Fayet, which has been manufacturing canes/walking sticks (a low-tech technology) since 1908, has designed the prototype for a 'smart cane', which is GPS-enabled and contains senses and software (in the handle) that allow it to track the user's location and build up a profile of their walking habits (McGoogan, 2017). The stick can connect with other devices to alert someone else if the user has fallen or needs assistance, making it a digital technology.

Digital technologies are crucial for mediating modern practices of care (Schillmeier & Domènech, 2010). As these authors point out, and as the above scenario shows, they allow for new subjectivities for 'care receivers', including people with a dementia (p. 3). One such subjectivity is 'knowledge maker'. Take, for example, how the latest study protocols for home-based trials involving digital technologies, outlined in Box 6.2, position people with a dementia and their family carers as knowledge makers. Most of these trials involve placing Ambient Assistant Living Technologies (AAL) into the family home, through which knowledge about a person's movements and care needs is created. AAL technologies aim to 'provide people with a dementia with the means to actively live their daily lives, protect their dignity, feel safe, maintain their capacities, sustain their integration with their communities and help their caregivers in monitoring and preventing unavoidable hospital admissions' (Novitzky et al., 2015: 709). We would, therefore, hope that if these trials were successful, AAL technologies would become more widely available to families who need them.

BOX 6.2 OVERVIEW OF LATEST STUDY PROTOCOLS FOR HOME-BASED TRIALS

1. TECH@HOME study is a randomised controlled trial underway in Sweden. It aims to recruit 320 dyads comprising of people living with dementia in a community setting and an informal carer. The intervention group will have a home monitoring kit installed in their home while the control group will receive usual care. The ICT kit includes home-leaving sensors, smoke and water leak sensors, automatic lights that monitor the individual's behaviour. Alerts via SMS and/or phone call will be sent to the caregiver should anything unusual occurs. The primary outcome for the trial is the amount of informal care support provided by the carer (Fänge et al., 2017).

2. Dem@Care is an EU funded initiative, which aims to implement a 'multiparemetric closed-loop remote management system solution that affords adaptive feedback to the person with dementia, while at the same time including clinicians into the remote follow up' (http://www.demcare.eu/). The study involves trialling a suite of digital systems.

3. The Easyline+ project (low-cost advanced white goods for a longer independent life of elderly people) is a collaboration between universities and companies in Germany, Spain and the UK to produce technologies that simplify an elderly or disabled person's interaction with a range of kitchen appliances, in order to allow them to live a longer independent life in their own home. The project focuses specifically on kitchen appliances as many accidents occur in this environment. Additionally, these appliances may pose significant usability problems for users with failing physical and cognitive abilities (Picking et al., 2012: 99).

4. The Ability-TelerehABIITation study aims to recruit 30 people with MCI or Alzheimer's Disease to an ability programme. The Ability Program lasts six weeks, comprises tablet-delivered cognitive (five days/week)

and physical activities (seven days/week) combined with a set of devices for the measurement and monitoring from remote of vital and physical health parameters (Realdon et al., 2016).

5. INDUCT – Interdisciplinary network for dementia utilising current technology comprises a wide range of academic and non-academic partners and technology in everyday life, technology for meaningful activities and health care technology (https://www.dementiainduct. eu/about).

The premise of most research into everyday (digital) technologies is that families or clinicians have a problem that digital technologies could resolve. The focus is then on the value of digital technologies to caregivers rather than the person with a dementia themselves. Take, for example, work conducted by a team of Japanese researchers involving the evaluation of a prototype ambient intelligent system that incorporated a smart carpet and door sensor, so carers could monitor the person with a dementia from a distance. Tests revealed that the system could effectively monitor persons, assess their activities and report the events online in real time, thus enhancing the caregiver's monitoring ability and mobility (Moshnyaga et al., 2015). Similarly, a small-scale study conducted in the United States involving five 'community-based dementia family caregivers' sought to investigate whether an E-mobile messaging service could reduce perceived 'caregiver burden' (Davis, Shehab, Shenk, & Nies, 2015). These studies, like so many others, prioritise support for family carers, rather than the person with the condition themselves. That is not to say carers are unimportant but that people with a dementia should not be sidelined.

Real-life stories of technological care and citizenship

To show what is possible when the care needs of people with a dementia are foregrounded, we recount two real-life stories of technological care and citizenship. The first is an uplifting story about one British man with a dementia, enabled to live at home with the support of his 'technically savvy' son Keith. The story appears in a report entitled *Technology Changing Lives*, which is about how to improve care and support in the community at a time of growing demand (Social Care Institute for Excellence, SCIE, 2015). Keith Spinks (senior digital developer for SCIE, and one of the contributors of the report) gives a personal account of how he supports his father technologically. Keith, who is visually impaired from a rare genetic eye disorder, is the main carer of his father who is totally blind, partially deaf, a type 2 diabetic and has a dementia. Reading Keith's account of distance caring, outlined in Box 6.3, we discover how comfortable he is using technologies and experimenting with different technological solutions to support his father.

BOX 6.3 HOW KEITH USED TECHNOLOGIES TO SUPPORT HIS FATHER AT HOME

When I found out that my dad had a dementia, I needed to know what the options were. In order to find that out, like any self-respecting geek, I went to Google. I entered 'total blindness and dementia' and I found one main reference that said 'care home' but I didn't think that was the right solution. I wanted my dad to live at home where I could help him get a care package. We have arranged three care visits a day and implemented a microenvironment. I felt that I could do a better job than a care home but there were still problems. This was in 2013 and as someone who has worked with technology his whole life, I found myself asking if technology could help improve this situation. So, I decided to try and find out.

I began by browsing the shops of the usual organisations, such as the RNIB, RNID and the Alzheimer's Society, to see what products were available that could solve my issues. What I quickly discovered was that nothing jumped out at me as a way to solve those issues. Unperturbed, I thought to myself where do I normally go when I want to buy something. As a man who doesn't enjoy shopping, I go to Amazon. So I went to Amazon and searched under dementia and I was staggered by the number of results that I got. What hit home was that I wasn't shopping in the right way. I was searching for solutions to problems that I hadn't actually identified yet. I needed to identify the problems that I was trying to solve in order to search for a solution. I could use Google, Amazon and other online tools in order to find those solutions. So that is what I did, and these are some of the solutions that I came up with.

The biggest problem that my dad had was that he couldn't find the toilet. Due to his blindness and dementia, he can't remember the route. To solve this, I bought talking motion sensors on which I recorded personalised messages to guide dad to the toilet, his armchair or the front door. It gives him an awareness of where he is in the house and when he moves across the beam it will call to him. As with all technology, there were many products that do the same job. I went through four different kinds of motion sensor until I found the one that worked well, which was cheap from Amazon.

My next problem was that my dad's sleep patterns were all over the place because he has no light perception, so he can't tell if it is day or night. I solved this by getting another talking motion sensor connected to the mains via a timer plug. This would play a personalised message telling my dad to go back to bed if he walked around at night.

Another problem that I encountered was that my dad would call me saying that he was lost or that there was a problem in the house. I needed to be able to see where he was and what he was doing. I bought four webcams and set them up at various points in the house and these can be viewed on my phone or computer. Now when my dad calls me I can log into the cameras and see what the problem is. One example of this in action was when I was in Dawlish, I got a call from my dad in London saying that he could hear an alarm and asking if he should call the fire brigade. I checked the cameras and could hear an alarm too. I worked out that it was coming from the freezer. This meant that I could reassure my dad remotely then contact the carer and ask them to look at the freezer when they next visited.

Then there was the problem of my dad telling me that someone, such as a nurse, had said something to him but that he couldn't remember what it was. For this, I needed another solution, which was motion sensor cameras. They record over seven days and if there is anything that I need to look back on I can review the footage. I don't have to do this very often, but it is there if I need it.

My dad's blindness coupled with his dementia meant that he was often hitting his head on things in the house. While the solution wasn't a technical one, I used technology to find it by asking myself who else often hits their head on things: toddlers. I found some rubber table edge guard usually used for toddlers and put it on corners, walls, edges and anything else my dad might hurt himself on. I solved a major health and safety issue for less than £10.

Everyone with a dementia needs a 'Keith' in their lives, i.e. someone who respects the right of a person with a dementia to live at home, and who not only understand the value of technologies but knows how to install and use them. Keith is digitally literate – that is, he is a competent and skilful user of information and communication technologies, who also understands how dementia affects a person's ability to function and use devices. The concept and practice of digital literacy is important here and is becoming increasingly important for people with a dementia to live at home; so, we will come back to it, in this chapter and the next, when discussing sharing responsibilities.

As Keith's story shows, for technologies to be accepted and used by older people (and their family carers), they have to be affordable and meet an identifiable need. One of the practical messages in the SCIE report, which is relevant to our discussion here, is this: 'start by thinking about the problem you are trying to solve, not about a specific form of technology. Then think through logically how you are going to solve the problem, using an experimental process with technology to find the solution that works for you' (SCIE, 2015: 3). In our view, the strongest argument one can put forward for using technologies is not so much a problem, but the idea of protecting and promoting a person's right to live at home. Rather than trying to monitor 'behaviours' or reduce the 'burden' of care for other people, we think more emphasis could be placed on upholding an individual's citizen's right to live at home. Although we do not know how Keith's father felt about his care arrangement, one can reasonably assume that he did not mind as he trusted his son to act in his best interests, and it meant he could stay at home.

The second real-life story features a Finnish woman, Lily, who lives in her own detached house, one half of which is inhabited by her brother, who is her carer. The story is taken from a research paper written by a team of scholars who recruited 25 persons living at home and diagnosed with Alzheimer's disease; participants were aged between 54 to 90 years – the average age was 79 years (Riikonen, Makela, & Perala, 2010). Lily (pseudonym) is one of the participants. This story, outlined in Box 6.4., shows how technologies can enhance care and citizenship.

BOX 6.4 LILY'S STORY

Lily lived in *her own household in a detached house*, whose other half was inhabited by her brother, who was her carer. The house was located in a *rural village community*. Lily had no family, but besides the brother her significant others comprised an aged sister, two nieces and her son's daughter. With the *progression of the syndrome*, Lily's use of telephone and contacts with the outside world had decreased; she had started to forget numbers. *Vendors at her door* had become another challenge, as Lily tended to trust everybody. She often spent weekends alone when her brother went to see a female friend in another location.

During the intervention, a *small size GSM camera was installed and home service visits arranged* to provide Lily's brother and sister some free time at weekends. The camera functions with a SIM card, along with a mobile telephone number that can receive images and video. The camera sends pictures and video to recipient mobile telephones or electronic mail at request by a text message or prompted by a motion detector using Multimedia message service or General packet radio service.

With Lily's agreement and at her presence, the situation was first *discussed with her neighbours* and other network member. It was agreed that the GSM camera could be installed above the house door at the top of the steps. The camera automatically sent footage to family members mobile telephones or computers each time the sensor had detected some motion at the door. *Whenever a family member became aware of visitors at the door through the GSM camera, he or she called the next door neighbour*, who went to see who was trying to enter. Lily's niece knowing when she was going to be alone, was able to pay special attention to those times. This arrangement *helped to prevent unwanted visits and to monitor Lily leaving the house.*

Taken directly from Riikonen et al. (2013: 237)

The story is a positive one. The whole intervention was 'needs led' rather than technology led, and it involved everyone concerned, including Lily, in the process of trying to find a solution to preventing unwanted visits. Moreover, it served to protect Lily's rights as a disabled citizen to live safely in the community.

However, we think the story raises several important matters related to the sustainability of technological care and citizenship, which we now outline.

The first is that the severity of a person's dementia is clearly a factor when using technology based tools and services. The habits and needs of a person living with a dementia obviously change as the condition progresses, as seemed to be the case with Lily, so there are judgements to be made about when, and for how long, technologies might be valuable for people with a dementia at home. Second, technological care and citizenship costs money and requires resourcing; in this case, Lily seemed to be in the privileged position of living in a detached house, which presumably she owned. It is not clear from the story who funded the equipment but it is reasonable to assume that Lily and her brother could have done so if necessary. Third, as the researchers of this study point out, a well-functioning social network is essential for the successful integration of technologies into a person's life. Installation of the GSM camera alone would not have helped to prevent unwanted visits and to monitor Lily leaving the house; her neighbour, family, professional care staff and the research team, also had a vital role to play. Fourth, consent to this form of care is clearly vital and was sought and obtained in this case. Lily was included in the decision-making process and would have presumably felt in control of the situation. However, it is not clear whether this was monitored at all.

This brings us to a final point we wish to make about this story in relation to the sustainability of technological care and citizenship. Lily's arrangement only works whilst this particular neighbour lives next door and is willing to fulfil the obligation, the devices and Wi-Fi connections all remain functional and each family member remains committed to each other and the arrangement. Any analysis of technological relational support needs to take account of these threats to sustainability and the duties and responsibilities that such an arrangement places on citizens, including people living with a dementia (Lily had to make a decision) – a point which we return to in the next chapter on sharing responsibilities.

Enhancing care

Technologies can enhance the care of people with a dementia living at home in one of two essential ways; first by supporting a person with a dementia to care for themselves, and second by facilitating others to care, including those living at a distance. Keith's story about his father's care arrangement usefully illustrates both of these enhancements, as it was the motion sensor cameras, which enabled Keith's father to get to the toilet by himself at night and allowed Keith to support his father at home from a distance. In this section, we discuss how various technologies, particularly digital technologies, are enhancing both self-care and family-care.

Let us consider first, how people with a dementia who still actively engage with technologies are using them to look after themselves. We know from our own research, on the use of GPS technologies by people living with a dementia, that the use of such devices can help a person stay safe. For example, a police officer easily found one participant after he got lost because he was carrying a location device. Other people with a dementia say they use everyday technologies such as talking books and earplugs to deal with the sensory challenges of the condition (Houston, n.d.). However, as we learnt in Chapter four, self-care is relational for people with a dementia; it inevitably involves other people. Thus, many people with a dementia are using digital technologies to care for themselves by connecting with other people with a dementia.

We are aware of many groups of people with a dementia, particularly across the United States and Canada, where distances between people are vast, which rely on the internet to support each other. DASNI started out as an internet-based support group; now people with a dementia are using video conferencing software such as Zoom or Skype to stay in touch, as well as Twitter and Facebook and other social media platforms. Using these technologies is a form of self-care, as they allow relations between people with a dementia to flourish. In a review of the literature on the experience of relations in dementia, researchers concluded that 'several studies emphasized the aspect of being with others with dementia, which could be an expression of equality, comfort or safety. PWD feel accepted as they are and are listened to and understood' (Eriksen et al., 2016: 365). Any technology that facilities this aspect of relation care is, therefore, an important one.

Everyday (digital) technologies can also facilitate self-care for people with a dementia who are no longer able to engage actively with the technology. In the same way, as health care technologies generally (such as transfer lifts and portable respirators) have made it possible for people with physical disabilities and illnesses to live at home, digital technologies have the potential to facilitate life at home for people with a dementia. This is important because as both of the real-life stories show, the outside world inevitably shrinks for many people with a dementia (Duggan, Blackman, Martyr, & Van Schaik, 2008). Life at home means just that for many older people with a dementia living with other disabilities and complex health problems.

For this reason, many researchers have focused on making the indoor home environment as safe and pleasurable as possible for people with a dementia with smart home technologies. Smart homes support the 'technological running of a household' through, for example, automatic lighting, infrared sensors to monitor room to room movement and recorded personal messages (Lorenz, Freddolino, Comas-Herrera, Knapp, & Damant, 2017: 4). In a way, Keith created a 'DIY' smart home for his father. Other people with a dementia might experience a smart home by taking part in a research study; then, we are likely to find out how the person with a dementia feels about the arrangement. For example, one team of researchers reported on a single case study involving an 85-year-old woman with a dementia living in a 'smart flat' within a sheltered accommodation scheme (Evans, Carey-Smith, & Orpwood, 2011). In this case, the person liked the automatic lighting system but 'started to feel constrained by the technology', which alerted staff when she left the flat (p. 251). This would suggest that even though the outside world may shrink for people with a dementia, individuals do not necessarily want the world to know, as and when they do try to access it.

For any technology to be integrated effectively into a person's life it 'needs to bring something of value to the person' (Pols & Moser, 2009: 166). The person using the technology needs to feel or experience its utility. As we have heard, some people with a dementia might like using the internet and social media because it means they can engage with other people with a dementia. However, people with more advanced dementia may need support with communication, and so a technology like Talking Mats may be of more value.[1] Reviewing the blogs on the Talking Mats website, it is clearly a valuable communication tool. For example, one 95-year-old woman with severe dementia used the Talking Mats app with her daughter-in-law and shared some things that she was not happy about, including her sore feet. Care staff were informed and a chiropodist appointment was made. In this sense, the technology enhances a person's ability to self-care. It also enhanced kin-relations, as the daughter-in-law and other relatives gained insights into this woman's thoughts and feelings.

There is often a fine line between whether the technology is of value to the person with a dementia or the family carer. This is especially true of older people with a dementia and more complex care needs. Take, for example, interview data from a qualitative study involving 13 people with a dementia and 26 carers, in which several people with a dementia said they used assistive technologies to keep their carer happy (Gibson et al., 2015). One person with a dementia 'accepted the use of a pendant alarm because she felt it helped her husband and main carer to cope with caring for her, rather than because of its direct benefits – the interviewer asked: How you feel about that, being watched via the pendant? To which the person with dementia responded: Ah, it's his way of coping with me. He cannot cope with the idea of me having dementia. He cannot cope' (p. 6). She recognised that the technology was bringing something of value to her husband and his ability to care, rather than her as an individual. An insight, which in of itself is significant, as it shows the capacity of people with a dementia to recognise the reality of technological relational support and to know when the responsibilities of care need to be shared – a point we return in Chapter seven.

Other researchers have concluded that it is not always possible to determine whom the technology is for. Maybe it is not even necessary. Instead, there is a constant negotiation of needs in terms of 'shifting between different perspectives: my, your and our needs for safety and security' (Olsson, Engström, Skovdahl, & Lampic, 2012: 106). An example is given in this paper of a carer who used a safety alarm to get help in an emergency when her husband had fallen on the floor, as she could not help him up by her herself. Clearly, in this kind of situation the connectivity of a digital technology can simultaneously benefit the person with a dementia and their spouse.

As well as enhancing self-care, everyday digital technologies can enhance family care. They can do this by helping the family carer to care for and about the person with a dementia as well as themselves. For example, in the Safer Walking Using GPS study, one female carer used the information provided by the tracking device to alert the police of her husband's whereabouts when he did not return home. There is a wealth of evidence that shows caring for someone with a dementia can be an isolating experience; just getting out of the house can be challenging for a carer if the person with a dementia needs round-the-clock support. In another study, researchers found that carers living in rural parts of Canada liked using video conferencing to form a support group, as it reduced travel burden and enabled them to connect with others in a similar position (O'Connell et al., 2014). This is where digital technologies can be a lifesaver.

Digital technologies are perhaps most valuable for distance caregiving. Distance caregiving whereby family carers live some distance away from the person in need of support is a recognised phenomenon (Benefield & Beck, 2007). Both the stories at the start of this chapter exemplify the standard practices of distance caregiving, which includes 'frequent contact with parents, mostly by phone; the establishment of arrangements with neighbours or close relatives; and keeping up to date with health-related matters so they could be informed when there were emergencies' (Collins, Holt, Moore, & Bledsoe, 2003: 310). The book *Care at a Distance: On the Closeness of Technology* provides a highly readable account of how everyday (digital) technologies, such as the telephone, webcams and wearable devices, are shaping caring relations between family members, and between family members and service providers (Pols, 2012). Although the discussion is not focused on people with a dementia per se, much of it resonates with this group, and so we would recommend it.

Enhancing citizenship

Technologies can enhance the citizenship of people with a dementia in several ways. First, by supporting people to grow and (re) connect with themselves and others; second, by helping people to exercise their rights and legal capacity; and third, by helping to position a person as a 'truth-teller'. Keith's story about his father's care arrangement illustrates each of these enhancements, as it was the motion sensor cameras that enabled Keith to support his father at home in a dignified way. In this next section, we review more of the technological focused research in the context of citizenship, meaning that attention is paid to how technologies support a person's right 'to live the life they choose and to be included in their community' (Article, 19, Convention on the Rights of Persons with Disabilities).

Technologies enhance citizenship by supporting people to grow and (re) connect with themselves and others. This is happening in multiple ways for people with varying degrees of cognitive impairment and previous tech experience. For example, an increasing number of people with a dementia are using social media sites (SMS) like Facebook, Twitter, YouTube and Instagram, to engage with others and talk about their lives. This trend shows the potential of digital technologies for enabling people with a dementia to be a 'good citizen', in that it entails a public display of concern for oneself and others. Take, for example, Peter Berry @PeterBe1130 who has Alzheimer's disease. Peter began a weekly vlog in June 2017, which at the time writing, he was posting onto YouTube and tweeting a link to every Friday. He says in one of the videos that his primary motivation for making the vlog was to help others learn more about the condition. However, he said he soon found that the feedback he received from other people helped him as well. Peter and others who are using digital technologies in this way (mostly younger people) are still in relatively good health and able to articulate themselves. For older, frailer people with a dementia, technologies that support leisure activities are perhaps more beneficial.

People with a dementia have a right to leisure time. Moreover, research shows that leisure activities can have a positive impact on cognitive function (Wang, Xu, & Pei, 2012). Several studies have looked at the benefits of gaming technology and Virtual Reality (VR) for people with a dementia. For example, in one study, 30 people living with a dementia were recruited from specialist day care services, as well as care homes, and randomly assigned to one of two groups to play a familiar game (solitaire) or a novel game (Bubble Xplode) at three different points over the course of a five-day period. The researchers found that people with a dementia could enjoy playing touchscreen games independently, regardless of the level of success that is achieved; the 'novelty of the experience seemed to be enough to facilitate enjoyment' (Astell et al., 2016: 1). Other work suggests that gaming technology might have a particular appeal to men, as it can help them to 're-engage with their old leisure interests' and promote a sense of personal growth (Hicks, 2016: 4). This PhD study, based on a sample of 22 men living in rural parts of England, is a particularly good example of how (gaming) technologies can enhance citizenship for people at home, as the approach taken positioned the participants as 'experts' in the development of this technological innovation (p. 191).

As well as gaming technologies, researchers are developing VR systems for people with a dementia to use. People experience a virtual environment through some kind of headset, which immerses them in a completely different place (like the coast or countryside). Researchers at Teesside, who wanted to explore how people navigate outdoor areas such as parks and streets, developed one of the first systems over a decade ago and demonstrated that it can be used by people with a dementia (Flynn et al., 2003). Since then, tech companies such as Tribemix have started to develop VR systems for people with a dementia and judging from users' reactions on the company's website, the experience seems to be a beneficial one. People with a dementia speak of feeling relaxed and revitalised, and one can see how it enables individuals to reconnect with themselves and others. In this sense, VR is not just creating a leisure opportunity, it is also facilitating citizenship-as-belonging. However, most of this work is with people with a dementia living in care homes, using equipment purchased by the service provider. This is because VR systems are not cheap – the Tribemix system costs over £4,400 – and so it is unlikely to be anytime soon before the average household has access to one. Of course, 'super rich' families could purchase one; one can even imagine a VR system becoming a technology of status and prestige (like iPads). Thus, some (expensive) technologies can expose or deepen social disparities.

Access is a disability rights issue. Not being able to access or use a service that other citizens (without a disability) can is unfair and may even be unlawful. In one study on the use of everyday technologies, it was found that 'people with cognitive impairment had significantly fewer relevant everyday technologies than those without cognitive impairment, reflecting less access to everyday technology' (Kottorp et al., 2016: 384). Digital technologies like Smartphones and GPS-enabled devices can be particularly challenging for people with a disability to access (Darcy, Maxwell, & Green, 2017). Not only are they expensive, others may misjudge a person's technical abilities. Thus, a person with a dementia may be given an assistive technology like a pendant alarm but be fearful about using it because they do not know what it is for – which is what happened to one of the participants in the study by Gibson et al. (2015: 7).

Technologies can enhance citizenship by helping people to exercise their rights and legal capacity. However, this is only likely to happen if a problem is conceptualised in terms of an injustice from the start. For example, the premise of the Safer Walking Using GPS study was that digital location technologies are a potentially effective measure to facilitate personal mobility and social inclusion for people with a dementia living at home (Article 20, United Nations Convention on Rights of Persons with a Disability). This is in contrast to the majority of previous studies, which start from the remedial position of aiming to 'reduce wandering' or 'reduce caregiver burden'. With a rights-infused approach, digital technologies have the potential to become a tool for promoting citizenship as well as care.

The potential of digital technologies for supporting the legal standing and capacity of people with a dementia has yet to be realised. Yet, this is an important capacity to support if we are serious about promoting the personhood and citizenship of people with a dementia. Take, for example, a woman with a dementia who Bartlett encountered during her PhD study. The woman told staff that she wanted a divorce after her husband moved her into a care home – a request that was not taken seriously. On the one hand, a lack of a response was perhaps understandable; it is a very complicated legal matter, especially if a person has been assessed as lacking capacity. On the other hand, not responding to her request indicates a lack of respect for legal capacity. As Gooding, Arstein-Kerslake and Flynn (2015) explain, the right to respect for an individual's legal capacity is rooted in the long-established right to equal recognition as a person before the law; to not recognise it is therefore extremely serious:

> Where an individual's legal capacity is denied and she is not free to make decisions in her own life, her opportunities to grow and change along with her environment and those around her are significantly hampered. Instead, she becomes a product of her environment, existing only at the whim of those who hold decision-making power over her. This may be a parent, guardian, conservator, social worker, or service provider. These substituted

decision-makers may have good intentions and may act according to what they believe is in her best interests. However, even a life that is good on the surface, but which is not led by the will and preferences of that individual herself denies the heart of the individual and creates barriers to the exploration and development of that individual's personality and being.

(Gooding et al., 2015: 243)

These authors recognise that people with a cognitive disability will need support to make a decision, and they suggest that assistive technologies, such as voice recognition software, and communication software, such as video conferencing, could help. In the above case, for example, the woman could have been supported to explore her options with a solicitor via the internet using screen enlargement applications if she needed to read information online.

Elsewhere, we have set out how technologies have the potential to enhance citizenship by positioning a person as a 'truth-bearer' (Bartlett, Balmer, & Brannelly, 2017). Here, we explain how technologies like the SenseCam – a device that is worn around a person's neck and automatically takes photographs when it is set to, has a potentially vital role to play in situations when questions of veracity are at stake (e.g. when best interests decisions are being made) (p. 1). Currently, SenseCam technology is used to facilitate reflection and memory recall for people with a dementia; however, we think it could be used to enhance citizenship by giving a people with a dementia a voice. Think, for example, of how valuable it might have been for Bridget (who met in Chapter two) to have had images of her encounters with the health professionals who visited her at home. She would have had evidence of the physically focused care to support her case for needing more mental health care. There would be weighty moral questions to work through, but this could have been achieved using an ethics of care framework. As we explain in this paper, 'the question thus becomes not whether we should use these technologies in the future or not, or whether they will bring about utopian or dystopian ends, but rather how and when we should use them within a given situation or relationship on a case-by-case basis' (Bartlett et al., 2017).

Conclusion

This chapter has sought to clarify and raise questions about the relationships people with a dementia have with everyday technologies. Everyday technologies have the potential to engender, in a person with a dementia, a sense of accomplishment or failure. Moreover, they have the potential to transform the way in which people with a dementia live at home.

Note

1 Talking Mats is a communication tool developed by researchers at the University of Stirling in the late 1990s to help adults and children with communication difficulties express their views. The original low-tech version uses a simple system of picture

O'Connell, M. E., Crossley, M., Cammer, A., Morgan, D., Allingham, W., Cheavins, & B., Morgan, E. (2014). Development and evaluation of a telehealth videoconferenced support group for rural spouses of individuals diagnosed with atypical early-onset dementias. *Dementia, 13*(3), 382–395. https://doi.org/10.1177/1471301212474143

Olsson, A., Engström, M., Skovdahl, K., & Lampic, C. (2012). My, your and our needs for safety and security: Relatives' reflections on using information and communication technology in dementia care. *Scandinavian Journal of Caring Sciences, 26*(1), 104–112. https://doi.org/10.1111/j.1471-6712.2011.00916.x

Pols, J. (2012). *Care at a Distance: On the Closeness of Technology.* Amsterdam: Amsterdam University Press.

Pols, J., & Moser, I. (2009). Cold technologies versus warm care? On affective and social relations with and through care technologies. *ALTER – European Journal of Disability Research / Revue Européenne de Recherche Sur Le Handicap, 3*(2), 159–178. https://doi. org/10.1016/j.alter.2009.01.003

Riikonen, M., Makela, K., & Perala, S. (2010). Safety and monitoring technologies for the homes of people with dementia. *Gerontechnology, 9*(1), 32–45. https://doi.org/ http://dx.doi.org/10.4017/gt.2010.09.01.003.00

Rosenberg, L., Kottorp, A., & Nygård, L. (2012). Readiness for technology use with people with dementia: The perspectives of significant others. *Journal of Applied Gerontology, 31*(4), 510–530. https://doi.org/10.1177/0733464810396873

Schillmeier, M., & Domènech, M. (2010). New technologies and emerging spaces of care – an introduction. In M. Schillmeier, & M. Domènech (Eds.), *New Technologies and Emerging Spaces of Care* (pp. 1–17). Farnham: Ashgate Publishing Group.

Social Care Institute for Excellence (SCIE). (2015). Technology changing lives: How technology can support the goals of the Care Act (June). London: *SCIE Report 73*, https:// www.scie.org.uk/publications/reports/report73-technology-changing-lives.asp

Wang, H. X., Xu, W., & Pei, J. J. (2012). Leisure activities, cognition and dementia. *Biochimica et Biophysica Acta – Molecular Basis of Disease, 1822*(3), 482–491. https://doi. org/10.1016/j.bbadis.2011.09.002

Wiles, J. (2011). Reflections on being a recipient of care: Vexing the concept of vulnerability. *Social & Cultural Geography, 12*(6), 573–588. https://doi.org/10.1080/1 4649365.2011.601237

7

SHARING RESPONSIBILITIES

Introduction: Why a shared responsibility?

The chapter begins by outlining why care for people with a dementia is a shared responsibility, and we suggest that certain shifts in the global policy landscape of dementia, and ageing more broadly, are making way for the idea of shared responsibility to evolve. Most notably the 'Dementia Friendly Communities' (DFC) movement, which seeks to include every sector of society, including banks and shopping malls, plays a role in supporting people with a dementia to live at home. This is one way of sharing responsibility. However, questions remain about the welfare of ordinary men and women with a dementia behind closed doors, who for whatever reason, do not benefit from the DFC movement. The sharing of responsibilities does not always just happen – although sometimes it can do. People may not realise or accept that they have a role to play. On the other hand, they may lack the opportunities and resources to do so. As gerontologists have noted, 'shared responsibility requires adequate opportunity structures' to facilitate it, especially in later life when support may already be diminishing (Kruse & Schmitt, 2015: 135). Thus, the second part of this chapter is about what it means to share responsibility.

Throughout this book, there has been a question about who cares for, and about, people with a dementia to enable social citizenship. Judging by the amount of attention given to family caregivers, it is apparent that the responsibilities of care and citizenship lay almost entirely with relatives, often women. It is a well-rehearsed argument that family members provide an enormous care service to people with a dementia across the world. *The Journey of Caring Report*, which analyses global long-term care trends for people with a dementia, contains an immense amount of information about the costs of home care compared to care homes (Prince, Prina, & Guerchet, 2013). The authors of the report concluded that 'the difference in the costs of dementia, from a societal perspective, between those with dementia cared for at home and those cared for in a care home are negligible when the costs of unpaid informal care are properly ascertained, accounted for, and valued' (p. 74). Currently, family members are shouldering the responsibility of care for people with a dementia at home.

Relying on one source of support is problematic though. It can take its toll on the caregiver. Taking sole responsibility for another person's care needs can be a thankless and invisible task for which there is limited support and understanding. Out of the nearly 1.4 million people aged 65+ in England and Wales providing unpaid care for a partner, family or others (Office for National Statistics, 2011), only 77,635 of these (in England) received any carer-specific support services (NHS Information Centre, 2013). This can lead carers feeling isolated and lonely, and when tasked with the care of another without help, stressed. In another report, by the Alzheimer's Society (2014), based on a survey of 1,000 people with a dementia and their family carers, it was found that:

- less than half feel a part of their community;
- 40% have felt lonely recently;
- only 47% said that their carer received any help in caring for them;
- 72% are living with another medical condition or disability as well as a dementia;
- just over half of people say that they are living well with a dementia – almost one in ten only leave the house once a month.

These data suggest that caring is hard work, and too much for one person to do alone.

A common rhetoric is that carers need to look after themselves to sustain their care responsibilities, but many family members must abandon the activities that help maintain well-being, such as working, fitness classes, attending the gym or socialising, to care. For example, the family carers who took part in our Safer Walking GPS Project frequently described their situation as time-consuming and exhausting. It was expected that they provide all the care necessary for the person with a dementia, often with limited support or help, 24 hours a day at home. One woman described having two hours a month to herself while her husband was cared for by someone else. The family carers described a lack of sleep due to increased activity at night by the person with a dementia. They had deep concerns about how they would cope if they were ill, as no one else was forthcoming to help. Looking to the future, they had fears about increasing care needs and how they would provide for them, as there was still an expectation that they would provide all care. External agencies may assume that these carers receive support to care as they attend, for example, support groups like dementia cafes, but it was actual practical help that was sought (Brannelly & Matthews, 2010). Supporting carers to care, in and of itself, is not therefore the whole solution.

Another problem with over-relying on family members is the availability of family due to work commitments or living away. Even though it might make sense for families to take responsibility, it may be that they are responsible for organising care rather than providing it. As scholars note:

> Many older people feel the responsibility for care should be with the family rather than with the state, although increasing numbers of divorces, more geographically disparate families, extended working life and increases in female labour market participation, will make such provision more difficult in the future, not only in high-income countries but worldwide.
>
> *(Kingston et al., 2017: 6)*

We are facing a watershed moment. As the older population growth is global, many counties face crises in supporting older people with a dementia to live at home. In the UK, austerity measures mean there has been a steady and considerable decrease of service provision, leaving older people without support. A social care crisis has arisen; there are 1.2 million older people with unmet care needs, and a 25% reduction in the number of older people accessing publicly funded social care because of tightened eligibility criteria (Nuffield Trust, Health Foundation and Kings Fund, 2017). Older people pay for care if they have savings above a small threshold and must organise care for themselves. For those older people and kin responsible for co-ordinating care, learning to negotiate care contracts has become the norm. Family carers describe this as time intensive, as it involves exploration of what is available, checking the reputation of care services, monitoring the quality of care provided, ensuring care that is contracted is provided and ensuring that the quality of care is adequate.

There is a societal expectation that family members will look after their relatives who have a dementia. Several qualitative research studies note how family carers assume the prime responsibility for the well-being of the person with a dementia (e.g. Orpin, Stirling, Hetherington, & Robinson, 2012). Health care professionals may be involved in a person's care, but the family carer has most contact with and knowledge of the person, so they take it upon themselves to provide all the care. This expectation can be very strong in some cultures. For example, in Eastern Mediterranean countries not providing support for elders in the family is viewed as a dereliction of duty and no dementia specific services are available (Yaghmour, Bartlett, & Brannelly, 2018). Similarly, in many black and minority ethnic communities, households may feel family care is preferable to using services, even though someone may feel like a 'bad person' when they find caring difficult (Moriarty, Sharif, & Robinson, 2011: 7). This shows how family members may feel under pressure to provide care even though they find it challenging.

Family carers are aware of what a responsibility it is to care for another person. Intervention studies, which aim to develop and evaluate education programmes for carers, have found this. For example, in one study involving

40 informal caregivers enrolled on a 7-week psychoeducational intervention program called, 'First you should get stronger', it was found that caregivers needed support regarding health responsibility, physical activity, feeding, moral development, interpersonal communication and stress management sub-dimensions (Lök & Bademli, 2017). These are considerable responsibilities for the average person.

Family members are not necessarily equipped to look after a person with a dementia. Very often, the effects of a dementia lead to a breakdown in care or some form of crisis. Crises are likely to arise from an unforeseen circumstance and may have significant consequences for the sustainability of a care arrangement. Ledgerd et al. (2015) identified five domains (see Box 7.1) that carried an increased risk of crises developing; these are behavioural and psychological, physical health, vulnerability, family carers and environment. The domains were based on the views of family members, professional caregivers and people who use services, and ranked according to inducing crisis.

BOX 7.1 FIVE DOMAINS OF RISK

Behavioural and psychological

Wandering such as wandering excessively around the home/outdoors and
     night-time walking;
Physical aggression such as hitting out and throwing things;
Sleep disturbance/excessive night-time activity.

Physical health

Falls;
Infections such as urinary tract infection and chest infection;
Delirium, confusion—sudden onset.

Vulnerability

Inability to identify potential risks such as leaving the front door open and
     responding to bogus callers;
Very poor eating and/or drinking;
Person with dementia being abused physically, verbally, emotionally, sexually
     and/or financially.

Family carer

Family carer burden through stress and workload;
Sudden absence of family carer for example through hospitalisation;
Family carer has physical health problems.

> ### Environment
>
> Physical hazards around the home;
> Hazards related to daily living tasks in the home;
> Living alone.
>
> Ledgerd et al. (2015)

Other research has shown that advancing dementia, advancing age and complications of coexisting conditions, makes care for people with a dementia at home by family alone an untenable situation. For example, in Brannelly's (2004) research of 50 people with a dementia whose care needs were changing, ten were placed in residential care, some unwillingly. Family carers were no longer able or willing to take responsibility for the risks associated with night-time wandering, unsafe cooking at home, falls, risks of abuse from neighbours, risk of aggression by the person with a dementia to others and the deterioration in a person's health due to a coexisting long-term physical health condition. More recently, researchers have found that family carers can reliably predict reasons for placement in care homes (Afram et al., 2014). This reinforces the point that relying on one source of support is problematic.

In sum, caring for and about a person with a dementia who lives at home is a shared responsibility. The changing and progressive nature of the condition and the multifaceted complexities of care it entails makes a single source of support inadequate. It is like expecting a lone parent to care single-handedly for a child with multiple disabilities. Alternatively, it is the equivalent to only one emergency service responding to a road traffic accident. Both situations require more than a single source of aid and support; they require responsibilities to be shared appropriately amongst relevant parties.

What does sharing responsibility mean?

The idea of sharing responsibility means two or more people or agencies having the same goal – namely, to enable a person with a dementia to live at home – and sharing decisions, costs and accountability in respect of that person's care needs and rights and duties as a citizen. As we have emphasised throughout this book, no two individuals or families are the same and so sharing responsibility is given meaning through dialogue and agreement between all parties concerned, including the person with a dementia. Fundamentally, it means that somebody is responsible for something and to somebody within the framework of ethics of care.

In the ethics of care, responsibility is a core tenet (Tronto, 1993; 2013). It holds an action orientation to create change and is instrumental. Without responsibility, care cannot be organised and implemented. It is one of the five elements of the integrity of care (described in Chapter five). It is also an identification of accountability. Tronto sees the ethics of care as the political process for enabling the ethic of responsibility. Drawing on Walker's ethic of responsibility, Tronto (2013: 53) argues that 'only through moral practices – the expression, agreement, and collaboration about the meaning of morality in any community – does moral life take form'. In this sense, responsibility is practiced and relational. In particular, working out the meaning of moral life and responsibilities is a continuing negotiation among people (Walker, 2007).

Collins (2015), in her recent attempt to summarise a core of care ethics came up with the slogan, 'care relationships generate responsibilities'. Responsibility seeks to make sense and create change through relationships, which are negotiated and dynamic. Interactions occur to create a responsibility; as Tronto (2013: 53) states, 'some form of relation – presence; biological, historical, or institutional ties; or some other form of "interaction" – has occurred to create a responsibility.' Thus, even personal responsibilities are shared responsibilities, as they have come about through an exchange of ideas and rely on cooperation. This is especially true of individuals and families living with a dementia, who share responsibilities on an ongoing basis about various matters.

Living with a dementia is a responsibility. It can take time and effort for the person with a dementia and their family to get a diagnosis and adjust to the idea of having the condition. Dementia can force people to seek legal advice and have conversations about potential future care needs and advance directives. It often disrupts long-held plans for retirement and growing old together. Unfortunately, specialist counselling for couples with dementia is currently difficult to find as therapists lack preparedness (Johnston & Terp, 2015). This is unfortunate as a diagnosis of a dementia can destabilise a marriage or partnership. Alternatively, and tragically, the responsibility of living with a dementia can become too much to bear for some people, and they take their own life (Wilkinson, 2015).

One part of shared responsibility is participating in decisions about one's life. Individuals and families have to make tough decisions and share personal information with health care professionals, even though guidance is lacking about the process of sharing decisions and responsibilities. For example, in a systematic review of shared decision-making, Miller, Whitlatch and Lyons (2016) found that there were various conceptualisations of shared decision-making with few explicit definitions used by service providers. Furthermore, the effects of the condition can change kin-relations and create discord amongst siblings who are expected to understand the challenges and come up with solutions. A single person and those without children may begin to rely on friends and neighbours for care and support. These changes can mean that sharing responsibility becomes an everyday occurrence for people with a dementia living at home – or at least it should do.

The sharing of responsibilities takes place within a policy context; these are the 'carescapes', which affect care exchanges (Bowlby, McKie, & MacPherson, 2010: 7). In Western societies, the focus of carescapes is often on personal autonomy, rather than sharing decisions and responsibilities. For example,

Barnes (2015) highlighted how 'care and protection' are placed in opposition to 'choice and control', where people who are viewed as able to have choice also get control, and if a person is not able to demonstrate choice and control they receive care and protection instead. This is problematic because people who need protection also need to have choices about the way their care is provided. Additionally, the wider network of care is at risk of being overlooked if the spotlight is on individual autonomy. This is far more likely to be achieved if responsibility is seen as shared rather than dependent on the autonomy of the person with a dementia.

There is evidence of divergence and change within carescapes. Not all national plans or international policies focus on personal autonomy. For example, Norway's Plan for a dementia-friendly society asserts that all 'sectors of society have a responsibility to ensure the equality of citizens with disabilities' before outlining the particular responsibilities that regional health authorities and housing banks have to people with a dementia and their families (Norwegian Ministry of Health and Care Services, 2015: 15). Likewise, the main recommendation in the Alzheimer's Disease International (ADI) report on the *Journey of Caring* is for countries to debate 'the balance of roles and responsibilities of the state, private companies, the third sector, and the families in providing care' (Prince, Prina, & Guerchet, 2013: 10). As well as policymakers, gerontologists are calling for more recognition of the 'shared vulnerability and responsibilities for care' (Grenier, Lloyd, & Phillipson, 2017: 318). Of course, none of this is easy. Care actors often have strong and conflicting ideas about what their roles and responsibilities should be, and then there is the big question of who is responsible for financing the care arrangement. Most debate, we would suggest, has focused on the economic question, rather than praxis about what it means to share responsibility, which is our focus here. Nevertheless, it is promising that the idea of sharing responsibilities is evident in carescapes across the world.

Who is responsible?

A key question in the debate about sharing responsibility is who is responsible – family members who live close by? Home care workers? Health care workers? Social workers? Neighbours and friends? Volunteers? Charities? Local communities? Police and rescue services? Community pharmacists? Churches, mosques and other places of worship? Grocery stores and other retailers and businesses? Of course, all of these agents have a potential role to play in supporting someone with a dementia to live at home. Indeed, the whole DFC movement, which seeks to include every sector of society, including banks and shopping malls to support people with a dementia to live at home, endorses this and is one way of sharing responsibility. However, questions remain about how and whether DFCs are sharing responsibilities and supporting people to live at home. In addition, who is responsible for the welfare of ordinary men and women with a dementia, who for whatever reason, do not benefit from or live in a DFC? Maybe they are housebound or live in poverty or a rural area. Who is responsible for supporting these people to live at home?

Care should be considered beyond the dyad (Barnes, 2015); to do this, the roles of all available actors are considered and made clear. Who is available will no doubt be dependent on locality; in some rural localities, for example, a few people may have multiple roles, such as neighbour and an alert for someone leaving the house unaided. In our Safer Walking GPS Project, police participants described how, in rural locations, the community act as a cocoon for the person with a dementia, alerting those who need to know about walking, for example, but also if the person had not been seen for some time. Strangers may be involved in care, for example, if a person with a dementia was lost and looking for home. Who takes responsibility also depends on the size of one's family and care networks; take, for example, Fiona and John, as outlined in Box 7.2.

BOX 7.2 FIONA AND JOHN DISCUSS WHO IS HELPFUL

Fiona listed the people who are helpful to her and John. They included their children, their consultant psychiatrist, Alzheimer's Society carers group, Forget-me-not Café (for the very valuable information they get there), sports memories workshops, Dr Gemma Jones for her useful and useable information, John's friends from the local Rotary Club and rugby mates, and friends at the camera club. Fiona and John are currently looking for some more stimulating activities to do during the day and are finding themselves considering things that they may not have done previously. Fiona was also considering getting someone to come and help at home but was unsure what to ask them to do – whether to do stuff with John or to free her up for her and John to do more together.

As we have already suggested, there is an assumption in any debate about balancing roles and responsibilities that family members take prime responsibility. It is often the case that relatives will rally around and do what they can to support a family member with a dementia at home. In larger families, like the Beek family – who featured in a case study analysis of care networks (Kruijswijk, Da Roit, & Hoogenboom, 2015), someone may need to take the lead for co-ordinating the care. As the authors explain:

> The Beek family is composed of six daughters, six sons and their ten spouses. After the mother passed away in 2007, almost all siblings and their spouses got involved in care of the father, who (had) Alzheimer's disease. Yet as the father's cognitive condition worsened several children stopped caring one after the other, until only six siblings and their spouses remained.

> Though the father needs round-the-clock care and professional care does not cover all needs, those relatives who are still providing care agree that he should continue living at home with their support ...
>
> ... In the course of time a 'core care team' has emerged around the pivotal role of Daughter-6 who has increasingly concentrated on tasks needed to keep the care arrangement running, like household management and planning of care schedules.
>
> *(p. 14–15)*

This is an unusually large family and so there are more relatives available to take responsibility. However, in this scenario, and we suspect many others, adult children stop providing care when things become too difficult – perhaps due to a parent's routine need for intimate bodily care, which is what happened in this case. What is common in this case, however, is the fact that a woman takes charge of the informal care arrangement.

Women provide a substantial proportion of family care to people with a dementia, with around two themes of primary caregivers overall being women (Erol, Brooker, & Peel, 2015). There is a lot published on the gendered dimensions of care, particularly in the gerontological literature (e.g. Kruijswijk et al., 2015). Some of which is beginning to filter through to dementia studies (e.g. Sandberg, 2018). However, what is most striking for a discussion about who is responsible for what is that 'women are more likely than men to help with the more personal aspects of care, such as bathing, dressing, using the toilet, and managing incontinence' (Alzheimer's Research UK, 2015: 7). In addition, 'women make up a large portion of the carers who are supporting someone with advanced dementia, who may be incapable of communicating or be confined to a bed or chair' (Alzheimer's Research UK, 2015: 8). This suggests that women take prime responsibility for heavier tasks for longer.

There are societal assumptions about who is responsible for caring. These are gendered norms, which tend to be biased against men. For example, Barnes (2006) recounts the story of a son who was caring for his mother. On multiple occasions, health care professionals questioned his suitability to provide direct care, despite the fact that he had worked as a nurse and a social worker in the past. Similarly, in our Safer Walking Using GPS research, it was evident that when a husband was caring for his wife, there was a sense that help would need to be more forthcoming, as it was less expected that he would cope. Furthermore, in families, where husbands were caring for wives, there was often more involvement from adult daughters. The point is that both men and women contribute to the care of people with a dementia at home, and it is important to recognise this (Kruijswijk et al., 2015).

Beyond the family, health and social care professionals have responsibilities for the care of people with a dementia. Questions about who is responsible for various care activities are typically centred on the family/professional carer nexus.

For example, Gilmour, Gibson and Campbell (2003) acknowledged the role that people with a dementia, families and professionals have in shared responsibility for assessing risk, and that resources and support are needed to achieve a sense of shared negotiated responsibility for risk-taking. Others argue that the responsibility for providing culturally and linguistically diverse communities in Australia needs to be shared across professional stakeholders for services to improve (Shanley et al., 2012). In addition, Iliffe et al. (2009) describe a shared responsibility for the diagnosis of a dementia between specialist and generalist health disciplines. This work is important, but it is based on a somewhat narrow parameter. On the one hand, it takes very little account of a person's wider care and support network (such as friends and neighbours). On the other, there is very limited evidence about how people with a dementia would like to share responsibility for themselves, or what shared responsibility may mean to the person with a dementia. People with a dementia do not seem to figure in the responsibility equation.

This is a significant omission. As we live interdependent lives, even if we develop increased dependency, we may still be responsible for providing care to others. For example, people with a dementia may well be a primary caregiver for another older person, perhaps a spouse who has more advanced dementia – as was the case for a husband with a dementia who took part in a study by Evans, Price and Meyer (2016). In addition, we know that younger people with a dementia still often have caring responsibilities for their children (see, for example, Roach, Keady, Bee, & Hope, 2008). Thus, the distinction of 'caregiver' and 'care receiver' is problematic, particularly from an ethics of care perspective (Ward, 2011).

Responsible for what?

Another key question is what are people responsible for – a person's health? Protecting a person from abuse or neglect? Caring for their assets? Responsibility carries with it a call to action to make a change. It is a response to someone in need and a recognition of need. Having responsibility denotes an acceptance of care toward another. Once responsibility is assumed, there are associated expectations from others about how the duties and activities of responsibility are carried out. Needs may be social, psychological, physical, spiritual and biological, and meeting those needs may require various skills, talents, knowledge and resiliencies. Multiple people may be involved in the indirect and direct meeting of needs, to provide hands-on care, to orchestrate care and to support carers – as we saw with the Beek family. Each person then has a devolved state of responsibility and are accountable for the actions associated with meeting needs. Often this responsibility is shared among many actors. Should anyone falter in their responsibility, it is likely that others will have to step up to take more responsibility, as irresponsibility is reckless and potentially neglectful.

Taking responsibility may mean the organisation of care activities but not necessarily the direct meeting of needs. Sometimes what is required is for

TABLE 7.1 Spheres of shared responsibilities

Sphere	Questions/Topics for discussion	Key (potential) actors
Information	What information needs to be shared? Who is responsible for sharing it? Who could find the information?	Person with a dementia; family; peer advocates; dementia navigators; befrienders; health professionals; state agencies; researchers; charities/third sector; interpreters; neighbours
Health	Physical health Mental health Sensory changes Identifying and managing pain Polypharmacy Abuse and neglect; use of screening tools	Person with a dementia; family, friends, doctors, nurses, Allied health professionals; community pharmacist; speech and language therapists; nutritionist, podiatrist; dentists; screening programmes; public health officials; interpreters; support workers
Social	Who is in regular social contact? What are their responsibilities? How much responsibility can they take?	Person with a dementia; family; neighbours; retailers; bus drivers; friends; family; inclusive cycling schemes; walking clubs; choirs; dementia navigators; befrienders; places of worship; restaurants; peer advocate; arts centres; cinemas, support workers
Legal	What rights does the person have? What practices are lawful/unlawful? How to protect legal capacity? Is there a statutory duty to care?	Person with a dementia; family; solicitor; charities; Citizen Advice Bureau; community police officers; interpreters, health professionals
Digital	Are digital technologies used? What are the desired outcomes?	Person with a dementia; family, grand/children; internet providers; telehealth workers, occupational therapists; peer advocate
Moral	What is just and fair? What are the desired outcomes?	Person with a dementia; family; psychologists; chaplains; faith leaders; counsellors
Cost	Who pays for what? What costs are reasonable?	Person with a dementia; family; public sector; regional authorities and municipalities; insurance schemes

someone to take responsibility for maintaining and promoting another person's independence – i.e. 'autonomy management' (Berry, Apesoa-Varano, & Gomez, 2015). Essentially, autonomy management involves supporting individuals to make decisions for themselves. However, it is not easy. One study involving 45 family members explored how people tried to share this responsibility but found it challenging; they said 'collaborative autonomy management work began to break down when family members saw affected individuals as unable to work with them to minimize risks' (Berry et al., 2015: 110). Some activities can become impossible to share, as and when the condition progresses.

A useful framework for thinking about who is responsible and what people might be responsible for is the idea of 'spheres of shared responsibilities', as shown in Table 7.1. We developed the framework for this text due to the lack of clarity and debate about the meaning of shared responsibility in relation to people with a dementia at home. When we consider care for a person with a dementia, family members and then professional care providers immediately come to mind, but it is helpful to consider the many others that help to maintain and promote a person's well-being. The spheres of shared responsibility framework facilitate that as it includes the more traditional providers of care (e.g. relatives) as well as less obvious people and newly emerging care actors, who are involved in providing care, such as public health officials and interpreters.

Each of the spheres of activity and groups of people in Table 7.1 may be considered for their role in the care of a person with a dementia. In fact, it would be useful for people with a dementia and their families to know who each group is, and the potential role they may play in the future – recall how Fiona and John (Box 7.2) wanted to ask someone to help them at home, but they were unsure what to ask them to do. In our Safer Walking GPS Project, one group whose role has increased with people with a dementia is community police officers, as they are likely to come to know people who go out walking a lot and who may be at risk of getting lost. Their role is primarily one of safeguarding the public, and therefore, any vulnerable person who they encounter is given opportunities for access to other services. However, the spheres of responsibility will vary across families, times and spaces; each situation involving a person with a dementia living at home will be different and shifting. Thus, the framework is best regarded as an adaptable tool for sharing responsibility, rather than a fixed model or approach.

Tools for sharing responsibilities

The sharing of responsibilities does not always just happen – although sometimes it can do. People may not realise or accept that they have a role to play. Therefore, it is helpful to think in terms of tools for sharing responsibilities – these are the mechanisms, frameworks and technologies for talking about and organising a shared plan of care and future care. For example, risk assessment templates and care planning tools are often used to capture and share vital information about a person's abilities and skills around the home. However, to our knowledge there are no such tools to facilitate the sharing of responsibility more broadly. Hence, we developed a new potential framework – i.e. the spheres of shared responsibilities.

A basic starting point for sharing responsibility is to write things down. Unless everyone knows what is meant to happen, no one can take responsibility for anything. People with a dementia and their families have a responsibility to share information. This might include facts about a person's background or details about their lifestyle. A Life Story Book is a tool that facilitates this – that is, a document that a person with a dementia is encouraged to complete with their family and friends before they go into hospital or long-term care. The idea is that by providing information about one's background, friends, pets and preferences, care staff will be in a better position to provide personalised care. Although a Life Storybook is not intended to be used as a tool for sharing responsibilities, we think it has the potential to be adapted for this purpose – but only if the spheres of shared responsibility are taken into account.

The advantage of recording the sharing of responsibilities is that the document itself takes on a responsibility. As science technology scholars explain, the documentation becomes a technology with the prospective of acting as an agent within a given situation (Latour, 2007). It does this by virtue of its materiality (its existence) and by joining together different actors, objects, concepts, ways of knowing and so forth, allowing them to take on quite different realities from place-to-place and over time (Law & Lien, 2012). Think of advanced care plans. In this way, the technology can take on responsibility for implementing certain actions and – to some degree – moral responsibility for the effects of those actions (Harbers, 2005).

Finally, we have indicated that the sharing of responsibilities can sometimes just happen. Some individuals and families will naturally share various caring responsibilities amongst themselves, without anything being written down. Take, for example, one of the participants – Chrissie (pseudonym) – in a wonderfully crafted PhD study by Barrie (2017). The fourth of nine children, Chrissie had a 'tough upbringing', which involved her mother leaving home when she was four and being quickly replaced by her stepmother (p. 129). For her narrative-informed research study, Barrie spends time with Chrissie, who lives alone in a terraced house in a former council estate in Scotland. As Barrie explains, 'Chrissie has three children, 11 grandchildren and six-great grandchildren, "*all less than a stone's throw away*" and she stresses that they are all "*really close*". "*We've all had our share of heartache, but it's kept us together*". This heartache includes the death of a son to alcoholism when he was in his late twenties' (p. 131). One of the activities that Chrissie really enjoys is going swimming at her local pool, but this involves various members of the family, including Chrissie herself, taking responsibility, like, for example, making sure she has the correct money for the entrance fee and telling people there that she has memory problems. See Box 7.3.

BOX 7.3 CHRISSIE AND HER FAMILY, SHARING RESPONSIBILITIES NATURALLY

Chrissie considers herself fortunate and imagines that things could have been different. Furthermore, she is 'still lucky' in having sons who keep the jars topped up, essential ingredients in a carefully coordinated plan that enables her to continue swimming in the future. Chrissie's imagining possibilities also include a time when she will not be able to drive, but she and her family are preparing for that. They are acting in concert; her sons are alerting younger family members to the demands made of Chrissie and her daughter is learning to drive, having previously had neither the need or means to do so ....

Chrissie would like a disabled badge and although it is clear that being able to drive and remembering where you park are unrelated, she won't apply as she feels this would be misrecognised as a sign of unfitness. Chrissie's concern with being identified as incapable extends to face-to-face encounters in public spaces and her fear of people finding fault is tainting the pleasure of swimming. Being with Chrissie illuminates the steps taken to negotiate the situation, including telling the woman at the desk about her condition. While this has the desired effect of no longer needing to produce her season pass, it comes at the price of being spoken to as if she is 'not the full shilling'.

Barrie (2017: 165/6)

This story shows how some families may already have the tools necessary to care for and about a person with a dementia. It is important for professionals to recognise and revere this.

Conclusion

Throughout this book, we have looked for ways that people with a dementia can participate in their care. In this chapter, we considered how others could help the person with a dementia to maintain well-being and be well cared for at home. Beyond the traditional idea of the care dyad, that includes a person with a dementia and a carer, there are many people who can be involved. We recommend that people are not left alone to care – that others are available to help sustain the person living at home with a dementia.

There is a crisis in providing adequate care for older people, and people with a dementia need resources to achieve good care. The increase in older people in our world is a story of the great successes of medical technologies and improved standards of living. But, as people age they are likely to encounter long-term conditions for which they require health and social care. Successive governments have failed to adequately prepare for the growth in the numbers of older people, despite knowing for decades that this situation would arrive. Hence, we find ourselves in a care crisis, where many older people face neglect because they do not have their care needs met due to a lack of adequate planning and political commitment to meeting the needs of older people. One of the shared responsibilities we have as a society is to ensure that people with a dementia are furnished with appropriate levels of support to live well and age in the place they want to. We would hope to expect the same.

References

Afram, B., Verbeek, H., Bleijlevens, M. H. C., Challis, D., Leino-Kilpi, H., Karlsson, S., ... Hamers, J. P. H. (2014). Predicting institutional long-term care admission in dementia: A mixed-methods study of informal caregivers' reports. *Journal of Advanced Nursing*, 71(6), 1351–1362. http://onlinelibrary.wiley.com/doi/10.1111/jan.12479/full

Alzheimer's Society. (2014). *Dementia UK Report*. Unpublished report. http://www.alzheimers.org.uk/dementia2014

Barnes, M. (2006). *Caring and Social Justice*. Basingstoke: Palgrave Macmillan.

Barnes, M. (2015). Beyond the dyad. In Barnes, M., Brannelly, T., Ward, L., & Ward, N. (Eds.), *Ethics of Care: Critical Advances in International Perspectives* (pp. 31–45). Bristol: Policy Press.

Brannelly, P. M. (2004). *Citizenship and care for people with dementia*. PhD Dissertation. University of Birmingham.

Brannelly, T., & Matthews, B. (2010). When practical help is valued so much by older people, why do professionals fail to recognise its value? *Journal of Integrated Care*, 18(2), 33–40. http://www.emeraldinsight.com/doi/abs/10.5042/jic.2010.0134

Collins, S. (2015). *The Core of Care Ethics*. New York: Palgrave Macmillan.

Gilmour, H., Gibson, F., & Campbell, J. (2003). Living alone with dementia: A case study approach to understanding risk. *Dementia*, 2(3), 403–420. https://doi.org/10.1177/14713012030023008

Grenier, A., Lloyd, L., & Phillipson, C. (2017). Precarity in late life: Rethinking dementia as 'frailed' old age. *Sociology of Health and Illness*, 39(2), 318–330. http://onlinelibrary.wiley.com/doi/10.1111/1467-9566.12476/full

Iliffe, S., Robinson, L., Brayne, C., Goodman, C., Rait, G., Manthorpe, J., ... the DeNDRoN Primary Care Clinical Studies Group. (2009). Primary care and dementia: 1. diagnosis, screening and disclosure. *International Journal of Geriatric Psychiatry*, 24(9), 895–901. http://onlinelibrary.wiley.com/doi/10.1002/gps.2204/full

Johnston, L., & Terp, D. M. (2015). Dynamics in couples facing early Alzheimer's disease. *Clinical Gerontologist*, 38(4), 283–301. https://doi.org/10.1080/07317115.2015.1032465

Ledgerd, R., Hoe, J., Hoare, Z., Devine, M., Toot, S., Challis, D., & Orrell, M. (2015). Identifying the causes, prevention and management of crises in dementia. An online survey of stakeholders. *International Journal of Geriatric Psychiatry*, 31(6), 638–647. http://onlinelibrary.wiley.com/doi/10.1002/gps.4371/full

Miller, L. M., Whitlatch, C. J., & Lyons, K. S. (2016). Shared decision-making in dementia: A review of patient and family carer involvement. *Dementia*, 15(5), 1141–1157. http://journals.sagepub.com/doi/abs/10.1177/1471301214555542

NHS Information Centre. (2013). Community care statistics: Social services activity, England – 2012–2013, table P2f 1c (December). NHS Information Centre.

Norwegian Ministry of Health and Care Services. (2015). *Dementia Plan 2020: A More Dementia-Friendly Society*. Unpublished report. http://www.alzheimer-europe.org/Policy-in-Practice2/National-Dementia-Strategies/Norway#fragment1

This involves acknowledging that a citizen with a dementia has a past, present *and future*, and given the right opportunities and support can live (and die) well at home. Using storytelling as a device, we have recounted various caring events and relationships, and explored how it is possible for citizens to live a meaningful life at home. We learnt of older men and women with advancing dementia living successfully at home because others recognised their right to do so. Each story in Chapter two mobilises the idea of respectful care, whether that is from family or home care workers. Moreover, the stories shared in this chapter and elsewhere in the book are testimony to the importance of taking the perspective of people with a dementia.

In Chapter three, the emphasis was on the progress and prospects for enabling people with a dementia to live at home. Here we took an idea from disability studies of enabling support systems and discussed the relational, service, environmental and structural components of such an approach to support men and women with a dementia at home. One of the most salient points from this discussion is to position people with a dementia as capable of exerting influence, as opposed to a 'burden'. Most of the research on life at home is concerned with reducing 'caregiver burden' rather than recognising and expanding the capabilities of the person with a dementia (and their family carer). Burden is negative and denotes a problem, whereas the 'language of capabilities refers to the real practical possibility of an individual being able to do and be certain things' (Venkatapuram, 2011: 115). Therefore, we prefer it.

In the case of people with a dementia living at home, capabilities might include going out for a walk on one's own, befriending another person with a dementia and maintaining contact with relatives who live some distance away. For someone with advanced dementia, who is completely dependent on others to meet their care needs, it is likely to be about the capacity to gesture and feel both pain and joy and all the sensations in-between. Essentially, a capabilities approach is about social citizenship; as one scholar explains, it is about 'choosing the life or being one values. While individuals are in the centre of this perspective, it has strong relational and indeed political elements' (Pfister, 2012: 214). Thus, enabling support systems to work at not only a deeply interpersonal level but also structurally – at the level of legislation, policy and strategic planning.

One area of growing policy significance is self-management. Governments throughout the world are urging people with a long-term health condition to look after themselves by, for example, taking regular exercise, watching what they eat and managing their symptoms. In Chapter four, we analysed the traditional conception of self-management and deemed it unsuitable for people with a dementia, primarily because it overlooks relationships. In our view, it is more appropriate to think in terms of relational care of selves; in that way the person with a dementia and those caring for them all become part of the well-being picture and merit care and attention. The importance of doing this became evidently clear when we considered how much people with both a dementia and diabetes have to 'self-manage'. Maintaining well-being and staying as well as possible ought to be the goal for people with a dementia and those who care for them, and facilitating this should be the aim of supporting organisations. Maintaining interests through adapted and supported activities, perhaps with the aid of technologies, is an emerging area of interest.

Towards a social justice agenda

The second part of this book focused on matters of social justice, including ethical and legal matters such as truth telling, access to and use of everyday technologies and the importance of sharing responsibilities between multiple actors. These debates serve to highlight the cultural sensitivities and complexities of living at home, and weightiness of moral decisions that individuals and families have to face on a day-to-day and nightly basis. In Chapter five, we explored the ethics of achieving care at home. This involved reviewing the research evidence on therapeutic lying and making the case for an ethics of care approach, whereby everyone states his or her needs. This, we would suggest, helps to create clarity about how to and whether it is possible to achieve those needs. In Chapter six, our attention turned to the technological aspects of care and citizenship at home. Here the emphasis was on the relationships people have with everyday technologies and how digital technologies can simultaneously enhance self-care and family care. In particular, we looked at the role and sustainability of digital technologies for promoting the rights of people with a dementia and distance caregiving. Like other researchers who we cite in this chapter, access to and use of everyday technologies is a matter of social justice for it raises questions about whether our caring responsibilities should change as technologies change.

The final chapter in part two explained how supporting people with a dementia to live well at home is a shared responsibility. After outlining the key reasons why responsibilities need to be shared, we focused on what it means, and how it could become achieved. An important point to emphasise here is that the sharing of responsibilities is not unidirectional. People with a dementia have responsibilities and are key actors in the sharing process too. For example, a person with a dementia may need to share information about themselves and engage with others; they may even need to take some responsibility for their own care (such as telling others what they need and do not need). In this way, the person becomes an equal citizen. As one leading scholar explains, 'citizens are not equal by virtue of being declared equal, but through an elaborate social process through which they become equal' (Tronto, 2013: 120).

A manifesto for improving life at home for people with a dementia

Our vision is for a society in which care homes becomes obsolete because the promise of sharing the responsibility of caring for and about people at home is realised. Our intention is not to rule out care homes as a long-term care option, but rather to embolden individuals, families, the third sector, businesses and government agencies in their endeavours to support people with a dementia at home. Everyone has a role to play in supporting people to live at home – from community geriatricians to the neighbour, the postal worker to the pharmacist, and supermarkets to sports centres and galleries. The 'Dementia Friendly Communities' (DFC) movement (for all its flaws) wants to recognise and facilitate this. As a civilised society, we have a collective degree of responsibility to enable people with a dementia to receive care at home.

We want the person with a dementia to have the final say in whether care has been achieved. Their views and opinions may need to be interpreted by others through the person's non-verbal and verbal communication. Alternatively, they may have an advocate to support them with decision-making and communication in the same way as many younger people with a learning disability do. In the future, we hope that digital technologies (such as face and voice-recognition software, and ambient intelligent systems) will have become so sophisticated and embedded into our everyday lives that they could 'read a person' and help them to articulate what they need. Similar to how brain-computer interfaces are currently being seen as the future for communicating with people with complete motor paralysis – or locked in state (Chaudhary, Xia, Silvoni, Cohen, & Birbaumer, 2017).

People with a dementia need to be taken seriously by their family members, as well as by health care workers and the wider disability and care community. We envision a time when people with a dementia are routinely positioned as capable of influencing and having a say in their care and treatment. When peoples' efforts to communicate are recognised and supported, rather than pathologised. We fear it is still the case for many people with advanced dementia that clear attempts to communicate, such as shouting and screaming, are attributed to the dementia syndrome, rather than the environment or an internal stressor such as pain (see, for example, Nagaratnam, Patel, & Whelan, 2003). This must change. We realise that the realities of life can often shift quite rapidly for a person with a dementia – for example, one moment a person may be annoyed about being confined to a space, but in the next, happy and untroubled (Moore & Hollett, 2003). Nevertheless, it is important that a person's legal status and repeated requests (e.g. for help, to leave, to get a divorce) are taken seriously.

We value our freedom. We value the freedom we have to move around, visit different places, express ourselves, take risks, change our minds and to write in the way we have done for this book. We think that each person with a dementia will have a set of freedoms that they value. Such freedoms are likely to be connected to the person's background and identity (e.g. the freedom to pray, or to go cycling or fishing, or to dress in a particular way). These need to be recognised and incorporated into life story work and advanced care planning.

We all have a responsibility. Each one of us has a personal responsibility to prepare for ill-health and isolation in later life the best we can. Yet how much time do we spend thinking about this? According to surgeon and author

Atul Gawande, not enough, as he points out: 'More than half of the very old now live without a spouse and have fewer children than ever before, yet we give virtually no thought to how we will live out our later years alone' (Gawande, 2015: 36). The problem is that some people will find it easier to think about and plan for later life than others will. Health and social inequalities exist. A lifetime living on a low income makes it very hard to take personal responsibility for one's health, as does living in an area with very high air or noise pollution. Thus, we advocate for an intergenerational responsibility to each other. This means doing what we can to make sure that the oldest in society are cared for well. Our care is not conditional on anything the person has or has not done, but by the fact of being alive, and because they most likely have been caring for others throughout their lives.

1 Professional practice

a.   We want assessment practices to change. Walking interviews are not the preserve of researchers; community-based practitioners could be using them as well to engage with people with a dementia who live at home. Some clinicians, such as Physiotherapists, Clinical Psychologists and Occupational Therapists, already go out walking with clients. However, we want to see walking and talking become a more routine assessment practice across the community sector with people with a dementia at home. This is because an enabling environment can only be viewed from the perspectives of people with a dementia and getting out with a person is the only way to see whether enabling environments work. In our own research, we were struck by how much more easily people with a dementia participated while being interviewed when they were out during the walking interviews. We know that other researchers have found the same (see, for example, Kullberg & Odzakovic, 2017; Normann, Asplund, Karlsson, Sandman, & Norberg, 2006).

Walking and talking is a powerful combination. In our experiences, it allowed for an assessment of the social connections and care networks that a person with a dementia has. Furthermore, it meant that the outside walking environments, such as buildings or paths that meant much to the person and with which they had a connection, stimulated the person with a dementia to speak candidly about their feelings. Part of living well with a dementia is the freedom to express, in the words of Philippa in Chapter five, the 'grimness' of it. We think it might be easier for people to do this whilst walking.

b.   We want professionals to care for and about all those involved with the person with a dementia, not only the person with a dementia or their spouse. In this way, there is a recognition that anyone who provides care is also in need of care. The idea of 'networks and chains of care' is useful here, as it reminds us that care events are linked to one another (Bowlby, McKie, Gregory, & MacPherson, 2010: 97). For example, live-in carers for people with a dementia are likely to have caring responsibilities themselves, but who cares for those who they usually care for? Live in carers are often economic migrants with uncertain citizenship in the countries where they provide care. This can make a person more vulnerable to exploitative working practices (Yeoh & Huang, 2010). Professionals need to know and care about this; otherwise, care arrangements are neither sustainable nor ethical.

c.   We want care arrangements at home to be reviewed regularly for sustainability and appropriateness, especially if they involve a technology (e.g. medications, sensor mats and GPS location technologies). People change, families tire, life moves on and technologies lose their utility or breakdown. We suggest that the ethics of care is adopted by practitioners to guide and critique reviews of practice. In this way, attention is paid to all the needs in a care situation, and responses are planned that enable those needs to be considered. This includes the needs of professionals, such as to uphold the safety of the person and provide care for their carers. The ethics of care can unpack care decisions so that is it explicit about whose care needs are met. When people with a dementia are taken out of this equation, care decisions favour others, or even systems over people (Brannelly, 2006). Thus, we think the ideal starting question for any review of practice is; what would make life good for you?

2 Education

a.   Educators have a responsibility to focus on the capabilities of people with a dementia and their family carers. It is important that the language of educators is positive and enabling, in that way people with a dementia and their families are represented as a diverse population. It has become popular to include people who care for people with a dementia in health care education, and increasingly people with a dementia are involved in teaching health professionals about their experiences. For example, members of the Scottish Dementia Working Group and Three Nations Dementia Working Group (all of whom have a dementia) talk to medical and nursing students, as well as others, about their lives. In addition, Bradford Dementia Group works in partnership with people with a dementia to deliver its specialist Dementia Studies programmes. This work needs to continue and be extended across the education sector for the wider care workforce, including, for example, general nurses, housing services, home care staff and police officers.

b.   We want to see more emphasis in education on technologies, and in particular, supporting people with a dementia to use everyday (digital) technologies that are important to them. As we explained in Chapter six, people with a dementia have relationships with technologies, as well as people. We therefore want to see a more focused effort on improving the digital literacy of care staff, so that they are in a position to provide technological relational care to individuals and families living with a dementia.

3 Care research

a. Funding bodies have a responsibility to invest in care research that will improve life at home for people with a dementia. Up until recently, most care research has been conducted in care homes. However, this is changing (certainly in the UK) as major funders in this field, such as the Alzheimer's Society and National Institute for Health Research, are funding studies that seek to support people with a dementia at home. We want to see funders invest in longitudinal studies that take a community-based participatory approach, as this involves working in partnership with local people, building on a community's assets and bringing about lasting improvements to people's lives.

b. Researchers have a responsibility to people with a dementia to report their findings as widely and in as many different formats as possible. We have discovered hundreds of excellent studies whilst researching this book, which have certainly convinced us that more could be done at a societal and policy level to improve life at home. It would be encouraging to see more home care research in the news and featured in podcasts, vlogs and public events. In that way, a much wider audience, including families, politicians and business leaders, could engage with research findings and see that life at home is possible.

c. We need to afford more control to people with a dementia in research studies. This means handing over some of our responsibilities as professional researchers to people with a dementia who would become citizen researchers. For example, we could train people with a dementia to interview other people with a dementia; work alongside families to help in the development of effective and affordable interventions for enabling life at home; and co-produce research outputs with people with a dementia, such as research papers, policy briefings and artwork. Whatever the activity, the process must be an equitable one.

Final words

Throughout this book, we have tried to stay close to the stories of people with a dementia and their families who live at home. Clinicians, professional caregivers and homecare workers have not been overlooked, but they have not been our primary focus. In so doing, we have prioritised the perspective of those who live at home and the relational aspects of care and citizenship. Life at home for citizens with a dementia is an ever-evolving achievement. We hope this text inspires you to do your part in realising that.

References

Bowlby, S., McKie, L., Gregory, S., & Macpherson, I. (2010). *Interdependance and Care Over the Lifecourse*. London: Routledge.

Chaudhary, U., Xia, B., Silvoni, S., Cohen, L. G., & Birbaumer, N. (2017). Brain–computer interface–based communication in the completely locked-in state. *PLoS Biology, 15*(1), 1–25. https://doi.org/10.1371/journal.pbio.1002593

Gawande, A. (2015). *Being Mortal: Illness, Medicine, and What Matters in the End*. London: Profile Books Ltd.

Kullberg, A., & Odzakovic, E. (2017). Walking interviews as a research method with people living with dementia in their local community Agneta. In Keady, J., Hydén, L.-C., Johnson, A., & Swarbrick, C. (Eds.), *Social Research Methods in Dementia Studies: Inclusion and Innovation*. London: Sage Publications.

Moore, T. F., & Hollett, J. (2003). Giving voice to persons living with dementia: The researcher's opportunities and challenges. *Nursing Science Quarterly, 16*(2), 163–167. https://doi.org/10.1177/0894318403251793251793

Nagaratnam, N., Patel, I., & Whelan, C. (2003). Screaming, shrieking and muttering: The noise-makers amongst dementia patients. *Archives of Gerontology and Geriatrics, 36*(3), 247–258. https://doi.org/10.1016/S0167-4943(02)00169-3

Normann, H. K., Asplund, K., Karlsson, S., Sandman, P. O., & Norberg, A. (2006). People with severe dementia exhibit episodes of lucidity. A population-based study. *Journal of Clinical Nursing, 15*(11), 1413–1417. https://doi.org/10.1111/j.1365-2702.2005.01505.x

Pfister, T. (2012). Citizenship and capability? Amartya Sen's capabilities approach from a citizenship perspective. *Citizenship Studies, 16*(2), 241–254. https://doi.org/10.1080/13621025.2012.667615

Tronto, J. C. (2013). *Caring Democracy*. New York: New York University Press.

Venkatapuram, S. (2011). *Health Justice: An Argument from the Capabilities Approach*. Cambridge: Polity Press.

Yeoh, B. S. A., & Huang, S. (2010). Foreign domestic workers and home-based care for elders in Singapore. *Journal of Aging & Social Policy, 22*(1), 69–88. https://doi.org/10.1080/08959420903385635

INDEX

abuse, concerns about 78–80
accessibility 48, 107, *see also* mobility
Admiral Nursing service 45
advance directives 74, 86, 117
advocacy organizations 59
Agile Ageing Alliance 33
Alzheimer's disease 1, 20, 34, 55, 81
Alzheimer's Disease International
    (ADI) 118
Alzheimer's Europe 74
Alzheimers Society 59, 80, 82, 113
Ambient Assistant Living Technologies
    (AAL) 97
anxiety 59, 61, 65
aphasia 19, 55
Arbor, A. 54
assessments 87, 132
attentiveness 84
Australia 44, 87, 121
autonomy 75, 83–84, 131
autonomy management 123

Baluchon Alzheimer's Belgium 43
Barnes, M. 78, 118, 120
Bartlett, R. 17, 19, 36, 94, 107
Bayer, A. 63–64
Beek family story 119–120
Belgium, studies in 43
Bernadette 24
Berry, Peter 5, 106
biographical disruptions 20
blindness and dementia 98–100
Boger, E. 57

Bowes, A. 78–79
brain games 58
Brannelly, T. 78, 79, 88, 116
Bridget's story 23–24, 29, 86, 108
Bryden, Christine 16–17
Bunn, F. 45

Campbell, J. 121
Canada 37
capabilities approaches 129
care 23, 85, 98–100, 105, 112
Care at a Distance (Pols) 105
care crisis 125–126
care ethics 7–8, 74, 83–86, 116, 133
care homes 3–4, 36–37, 79–80, 106,
    130–131, *see also* institutionalization
Care of Persons with Dementia in their
    Environments (COPE) 43
care research 134
caregiver burden 16, 36–38, 43, 98, 113,
    115, 129
caregiver perspectives 93–94, 98
caregiver/recipient dynamics 43, 79, 121
carers 8, 73, 75, 79, 85, 104, 113
carescapes 117–118
China 48–49
Chrissie's story 124–125
citizenship 2–3, 15–16, 19, 38, 105–106,
    130, *see also* social media
cognitive decline 63
cognitive function 106
cognitive training 58
collectivism 54, 66

Collins, S. 117
communication 104, 131
communities of care 66, 67, *122*, 123
community-based services 4, 33, 43, 45
complications, of multiple conditions 57
confinement 47–48
Connecticut Home Care Program For
 Elders 43
control 39–40, 44, 46, 60–61, 118
Creutzfelt-Jacob disease 55
crises, and care arrangements 115–116
cultural norms 4, 10, 26, 45, 114

Daniel, B. 78–79
Day, A. M. 78
deceptive practices. *see* therapeutic lying
decision-making: and conflict 85–86;
 ethical 83–86; family domination of
 7, 34; for the future 86; inclusion in 2,
 18, 27–28, 39–40, 61–62, 64, 86–87,
 102; and information 61; and mental
 capacity 87; process 61–62, 86; by
 proxy 87
Dem@Care 94, 97
dementia 55; defining 34, 55;
 diagnosis impacts 117; diagnosis
 overtaking identity 7, 34, 62, 64,
 88; differing lived experiences 16;
 and environmental demands 46; and
 other long-term health conditions 35,
 57; statistics 1, 15, 63; symptoms 55,
 62–63, 77; terms used for 9
Dementia Action Alliance 18
Dementia Advisors 27–28
dementia diagnosis, issues raised by 74–75
Dementia Diaries 5, 17
Dementia Dogs program 42
Dementia Friendly Communities (DFC)
 11, 49, 112, 118–119, 131
dementia patients, rights of 3–4, 11,
 18–19, 42, 61, 64, 87–88, 93–94, 105,
 107, *122*, 130
Dementia Statements 18
democratic spaces 46
Denmark 96
diabetes 35, 56, 62–65
digital literacy 100
disability, defining 34
domestic maids 9

early-onset dementia 20, 80, 81, 96
EasyLine+ project 97
education, and dementia 133–134
enabling: defining 32; environmental
 45–48; and familiarity 46;

relational 38–42; service-level 42–45;
 structural 48–50
enabling support systems 33, *35*, 38
end-of-life care 75
environmental demands 46
environmental enabling 45–48
environmental risks 116
Equality Act 18
ethical issues of dementia 74–76
ethics of care 7–8, 66, 74, 83–86,
 116, 133
Evans, D. 40

familiar environments, limitations of 46
families: and care relationships 18,
 22, 43, 54, 60–62, 104, 112–113,
 119–121, *see also* relationships; shared
 responsibilities; *specific stories*
Farsides, B. 81
feeling out of place 16, 47
filial piety 26, 45
Fiona and John 58–59, 65–66, 119, 123
flexible care arrangements 43
Frank, Arthur 16, 19–20, 21
freedom 131
frontal-temporal lobe dementia 34, 55,
 73, 80–81
Fulda, K. G. 82
functional ability 34–35

Gawande, Atul 131–132
gender 7, 40, *see also* men; women
gender/sexuality, importance of 28
genetic testing 73, 80–83
Geriant model of care 45
Germany 35, 44
gerontechnology 3
Gibson, F. 121
Gilligan, Carol 7–8
Gilmour, H. 121
good care 74
GPS 75, 86, 103, 107
grief, caregiver's 27

Hamed's story 47
happiness, factors for 42
Hayata, Masami 25–26, 29
health-care focus 25
health professionals 56–57, 75
health services, vs. support groups 57
healthy lifestyles, and dementia impacts
 58, 62
Hellström, I. 44
hidden disabilities 34
Hilison, R. 63–64

Holman, H. R. 56
home care 21–22, 24–25, 27
hospitals: admission trends 22; assessments
    in 37; and decision-making 87;
    destabilising factors 46
Huntington's Chorea 55, 73, 81–82

Iceland 49–50
idealised lifestyles 57
Iliffe, S. 121
incontinence 36
independence, importance of 54
India 48
INDUCT study 98
information 44, *122*
institutionalization 3, 36–37, 43, 49–50,
    60, 79–80, *see also* care homes
integrated care 45
interconnectivity 8
International Human Rights law 18
interpersonal relationships, and
    caregiving 2

Jair, Sion 47
James, I. A. 78
Japan 25–26, 79, 98
John's story 58–59, 65–66, 119
Journey of Caring Report 112–113, 118

Karen and Martin's story 94
Keith's story 98–100, 105
Kirk, J. K. 56
Kishimoto, Y. 79
Kitwood, Tom 38
knowledge-makers 97
Kwok, J. B. J. 81

lack of control, studies of 39
Larsson, A. 44
Ledgerd, R. 115
Lee, D. R. 78
legal capacity/rights 107–108, *122*, 129
Lewy Body dementia 55
life expectancy, in the UK 4
Life Story Books 124
Lily's story 101–102
live-in carers 22–23, 43–44, 132–133
living alone: challenges of 40; and
    institutionalization 37; technological
    mishaps 95–96; and technology 93,
    99–102; together 40–41
loneliness 41–42
long-distance care 23, 98–100, 105
Lorig, K. 56
Loy, C. l. 81

lying. *see* therapeutic lying
Lykens, K. 82
Lyons, K. S. 117

Malcolm and Nigel's story 26–28
Māori culture 66
marginalization 7–8, 28, 84
memory aids 93, 95
memory cafes 44
memory training 57
men: as carers 25–26, 29, 98–100, 104,
    120, *see also* spousal responses
mental capacity, assessing 87
Mental Capacity Act (2005) 87, 88
Mental Capacity Act Best Interest
    Meetings 27
Meyer, J. 40
Meyer, T. D. 78
migrant care workers 9, 22–23, 133
migrants 45
Miller, L. M. 117
MindMate 95
Mini-Mental State Examination 63
mini-strokes, instead of dementia
    diagnosis 23, 25
minority communities 44–45, 114
Mitchell, Wendy 16
mixed dementia 55
mobility 47, *see also* accessibility
monitoring techniques 75

national plans for dementia 49
negative stereotypes 17, 60
Netherlands 45–46
Nigel and Malcolm's story 26–28
Norway 39, 118
*Nuffield Council on Bioethics, Dementia:
    Ethical issues* 83
nursing homes. *see* care
    homes; institutionalization

Odensehuis 46
On Our Radar 5

paid carers: live-in 22–23, 43–44; long
    term relationships with 24, 25, 29; pay
    rates 8, 22; and therapeutic lying 78;
    training levels of 22
palliative care 75, 86
Parkinson's Disease 55
participative inquiry 6
Paulsen, J. S. 82
peer support 41
personal assistants 43–44
personhood 84

pets 41–42
Phillipa 73, 76–77, 78, 80–81
Picks Disease 34, 55, 73, 80–81
Piette, J. D. 54
place: defining 47, *see also*
    familiar environments
poetry 20
police officers 123
Pols, J. 105
polypharmacy 57
Posterior Cortical Atrophy (PCA) 34
power of attorney 74, 86
Pratchett, Terry 34
Price, K. 40
problems, identifying 99, 100
Protection of the Rights and Interests of
    the Elderly People (2013) 48–49
protection vs. control 118
public transportation 48

Raglan Project 25
recognition 44–45
relational care 65, 129–130
relational enablers 38–42
relational living 38–39
relationship-centred approach to care
    25, 101
relationships 29, 41, 65, 75, 104,
    see also families
research 134; demand for 1; into
    technology 103–104; missing
    perspectives in 64; tendencies in 33
responsibilities: defining 121, 123; of
    families 112–115; sharing 2, 116–121,
    122, 123, 130
responsibility: and caring 84; and
    self-management 57, *58*, 59
RightTimePlaceCare study 36
risk assessment templates 123–124
risks 60–61, 115–116, 123–124
Roberts, S. J. 81, 82
rural locations 119

Safer Walking GPS Project 6, 41–42, 48,
    59–60, 65, 86, 96, 105, 113, 120, 123
Schofield, P. R. 81
Scottish Dementia Working Group 133
Seaman, A. T. 77
self-management 56, 129; criticisms
    56–57; and decision-making 61–62;
    defining 1–2, 10, 54, 55; drawbacks of
    10, 65, 67; and quality of life 64; and
    technology 103; traits of 57–62
Senior Citizens Act (2007) 48
Seniors in Transition study 37

SensCam 108
service animals 42
service-level enabling 42–45
sexuality 28
shared responsibilities 116–121, *122*,
    123–124, 130
shrinking worlds 23–24, 47–48,
    60, 103–104
Sinclair, A. 63–64
Singapore 44
smart homes 103
Smebye, K. L. 80
social media 5, 103, 105
soft paternalism 80
solidarity 85
spheres of shared responsibilities *122*, 123
spousal responses 17, 18, 22, 37, 40
stability 35–36, 47
statistics: dementia rates 1, 63; on
    dependency 25; diabetes 62–63;
    institutionalization 3, 43, 49; living
    at home with dementia 15; multiple
    health conditions 35; primary carers
    26; unpaid care 113; widows/
    widowers 23
Stone, A. M. 77
Strech, D. 75
structural enabling 48–50
suicide 117
support 41–42, 59, 99–100
support groups 16, 20, 57, 80, 105, 113
support needs 37, 113–114
support services 16, 43
support systems 33–34, 39
Swaffer, Kate 16–17
Sweden 44, 45, 47

Talking Mats 104, 108*n*1
Talking Point forum 60
Taller Than the Trees (Mylan) 25–26, 29
Tasmania 44
Tech@Home study 97
technology 11, 97–98, 108, 133; for
    communication 104; defining 92;
    digital 96–97, 98, 103, 130; and living
    alone 93, 99–100; mishaps with 22, 95,
    95–96; monitoring 98; perceptions of
    93, 104, 107; relationships with 92–93,
    95, 102–104; virtual reality 106; and
    vulnerability 96, *see also* GPS
Technology Changing Lives report 98–100
therapeutic lying 11, 75–78
Three Nations Dementia Working
    Group 133
triangle of care model 92

Tronto, Joan 7–8, 84–85, 116–117
trust 11, 24, 76–78
truth-telling 73, 76–77, 105, 130
Turner, A. M. 81

Uhlmann, W. R. 81, 82
United Kingdom: Admiral Nursing
  service 45; Dementia Action Alliance
  18; Dementia Friendly Communities
  49; institutionalization 50; life
  expectancy 4; Mental Capacity Act
  (2005) 87–88; public transportation
  48; studies in 4; support costs 114; and
  technology 96; widows/widowers 23
United States, studies in 17, 43

vascular dementia 26, 55
violence 36–37, 73, 78–80, 83, 116
virtual reality (VR) technology 106
voice recognition software 92
vulnerabilities 96, 115

walking interviews 132
Western values 10
whānau 9, 66
Whitlach, C. J. 117
William's story 21–23, 29, 95
women, and care responsibilities
  112, 120
Work Package (RightTimePlaceCare
  study) 36

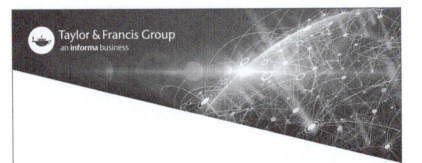